33

33
...

Dr. David Serio

© 2017 Dr. David Serio
All rights reserved.

ISBN-13: 9781977783233
ISBN-10: 1977783236

Contents

Contributors · ix
Forward · xi
Introduction · xv
Disclaimer · xvii
My Journey · xix

Principle 1   The Major Premise · 1
              Dr. Arno Burnier
Principle 2   The Chiropractic Meaning of Life · · · · · · · · · · · · · · · · 8
              Dr. Bill Decken
Principle 3   The Union of Intelligence and Matter · · · · · · · · · · · · · 15
              Dr. Gilles A. LaMarche
Principle 4   The Triune of Life · 21
              Dr. Mark Romano
Principle 5   The Perfection of the Triune · · · · · · · · · · · · · · · · · · 27
              Dr. Stamatis Tsamoutalidis
Principle 6   The Principle of Time · 35
              Dr. Joe Donofrio and Dr. Mark Romano
Principle 7   The Amount of Intelligence in Matter · · · · · · · · · · · · · 42
              Dr. Autumn Hicks Gore
Principle 8   The Function of Intelligence · · · · · · · · · · · · · · · · · · 47
              Dr. Christopher Kent
Principle 9   The Amount of Force Created by Intelligence · · · · · · · · · 55
              Dr. Judy Nutz Campanale

Principle 10	The Function of Force · 62	
	Dr. Shane Walker	
Principle 11	The Character of Universal Forces · · · · · · · · · · · · · · · · · · 68	
	Dr. Edwin Cordero	
Principle 12	Interference with Transmission of Universal Forces · · · · 73	
	Dr. Caroline Lagerlof	
Principle 13	The Function of Matter · 80	
	Dr. Pam Jarboe	
Principle 14	Universal Life · 87	
	Dr. Sophie Anderson	
Principle 15	No Motion without the Effort of Force · · · · · · · · · · · · · · 94	
	Daniel Facchini, Chiropractor	
Principle 16	Intelligence in both Organic and Inorganic Matter · · · · 100	
	Dr. Joseph B. Strauss	
Principle 17	Cause and Effect · 109	
	Dr. Lona Cook	
Principle 18	Evidence of Life · 115	
	Dr. Phil McMaster	
Principle 19	Organic Matter · 122	
	Dr. Eric Russell	
Principle 20	Innate Intelligence · 129	
	Dr. Steve Tullius	
Principle 21	The Mission of Innate Intelligence · · · · · · · · · · · · · · · · · 136	
	Dr. Patty Cosmelli	
Principle 22	The Amount of Innate Intelligence · · · · · · · · · · · · · · · · · 141	
	Dr. Kim R. Stetzel and Greg A. Stetzel	
Principle 23	The Function of Innate Intelligence · · · · · · · · · · · · · · · · 149	
	Dr. Simon Senzon	
Principle 24	The Limits of Adaptation · 154	
	Dr. Peter Kevorkian	
Principle 25	The Character of Innate Forces · · · · · · · · · · · · · · · · · · · 160	
	Dr. Sharon Gorman	
Principle 26	Comparison of Universal and Innate Forces · · · · · · · · · · 166	
	Dr. Richard Grostic	

Principle 27	The Normality of Innate Intelligence ················ 175	
	Dr. Andreas Soderstrom	
Principle 28	The Conductors of Innate Forces ·················· 180	
	Dr. Andy Roberts	
Principle 29	Interference with the Transmission of Innate Forces ··· 186	
	Dr. Dan Sullivan	
Principle 30	The Causes of Dis-ease ························· 191	
	Dr. Kari Swain	
Principle 31	Subluxations ································· 198	
	Dr. Rob Sinnott	
Principle 32	The Principle of Coordination ···················· 205	
	Dr. Liam Schubel	
Principle 33	The Law of Demand and Supply ··················· 211	
	Dr. Lacey Book and Shawn Dill	
	Acknowledgments ······························ 225	
	About the Author ······························ 227	

Contributors

Forward	Dr. Thom Gelardi
Introduction	Dr. David Serio
My Journey	Dr. David Serio
Our Time Has Come	Dr. David Serio
Practice Pre-Game	Dr. David Serio
Tonality	Dr. David Serio
KISS	Dr. David Serio
Appreciation and Attraction	Dr. Richelle and Daniel Knowles
Adding Value through Education and Communication	Dr. David Serio
Our Craft	Dr. Damaris-Leigh Lanjopolous
Success Formula	Sebastian Carera Chiropractor
Simplicity	Dr. Mary Hellen Hensley
A Peak into the Mind of a Chiropractic Professor	Dr. Brian Dooley
Certainty of Truth	Dr. Chris Zaino
To Give, To Do, To Love, To Serve	Dr. David Serio
Practice Management by Objective	Dr. David Serio
Servants Heart	Dr. Christopher Wolff
Love What you Do and Do What you Love	Dr. David Serio
Levels of Conciousness	Jane Burnier Life Coach and CA
Explode your Practice	Dr. Steve Judson
Signs of Life	Dr. Joe Donofrio

The Bigness of Chiropractic	Dr. Arno Burnier
Build a Chiropractic Dynasty	Dr. David Serio
Present Time Conciousness	Dr. David Serio
Success in Practice	Dr. Thomas Waller
Your Internal GPS	Dr. David Serio
Relationship and Connection	Dr. David Serio
Futurism and Thriving	Dr. David Serio
Transformation	Dr. Daniel R. Constable
Crush your Comfort Zone	Dr. David Serio
Craft	Dr. David Serio
Choices	Dr. David Serio
The Four Levels of Influence	Dr. David Serio
Sacred Trust	Dr. BJ Palmer
Bonus: Blue Ocean Marketing Strategy	Dr. Andreas Soderstrom

Forward
Thomas A. Gelardi, DC

• • •

THE WORLD IS ABUZZ LIKE never before. It is being hailed as the greatest advance in health care since William Harvey's discovery of the circulatory system. Some are saying that the Noble Prize is insufficient for recognizing the magnitude of this rediscovery. It is rumored that the United Nations is considering a $1 billion prize, claiming $1 million would be a mere pittance compared to the trillions of dollars the world will save, annually, from its programs developing new vaccines, blood thinners, painkillers, antibiotics, antidepressants, anti-inflammatories, and a host of other pharmaceuticals. It will also alleviate much associated suffering and reduce hospital stays and office visits, it claims. Lives will be more vibrant, creative, and well lived.

As happens rarely, this great scientific breakthrough was not made by teams of scientists working in university laboratories. Like Einstein's discovery of the special and general theories of relativity and the concept of mass-energy equivalence expressed through his most famous equation, $E=mc^2$, this rediscovery also took place outside the laboratory and through the human intellect and imagination alone.

The latest rediscovery, articulated by Matthew, took place about two thousand years ago and was recorded in the King James Version of the Bible under Matthew 7:14. An original discovery is known to have taken place much earlier, but scholars do not agree as to the era. Again, similar to Einstein and other theoretical physicists, Matthew used material metaphors to explain his nonmaterial ideas.

Matthew's statement has never had more and greater practical applications in the area of health than it does today, with all its unnatural lifestyles and manufactured toxins. It is a world changer. It is stated simply and powerfully as, "Strait is the gate, and narrow is the way, which leads unto life, and few there be that find it." I assume he believed that most people could find it if they chose.

Mathew's dictum is as true today as it was two thousand years ago, and it will be true as long as the universe continues to operate according to universal law. We have no choice about obeying universal law. Everyone and everything obeys universal law. Our only choice is in deciding where we want to go in life and which universal laws will get us there. Ella Wheeler Wilcox expressed that idea in her metaphorical poem "'Tis the Set of the Sail." It includes the following stanza:

> One ship sails East,
> And another West,
> By the self-same winds that blow,
> 'Tis the set of the sails
> And not the gales,
> That determine where they go.

Dr. Serio's book is especially helpful for those in search of optimum, autonomous physical, emotional, and spiritual health. The ancients knew that they who had health had everything, including social and financial well-being. His book also is for the merely curious. I have discovered much of value during curious excursions.

Those who knowingly or unknowingly use universal law for constructive purposes are enhanced in every area of their lives, and all other lives are enhanced. Those who knowingly or unknowingly use universal law for destructive purposes are injured and suffer, and all other lives are injured and suffer. "When we try to pick out anything by itself, we find it hitched to everything else in the universe," wrote John Muir, the Sierra Club founder.

A few last words. This is a philosophy book; it explains the principles underlying the chiropractic's central area of interest. Philosophy takes into account all information, including current concepts from material science, as well as nonmaterial concepts, such as life, health, values, and wisdom, generally considered by philosophy. I recommend that you study these principles and then consider them in relation to the expression of all forms of life and to health in just the physiological area. Question everything and I highly recommend studying this book with others.

Introduction
Dr. David Serio

• • •

FOR YEARS I ASKED MYSELF, *what are the characteristics that successful, long-lasting corporations, cultural movements, people, and professions have in common? What I discovered is that they have a razor-sharp mission combined with a clear, well-thought-out philosophical construct guiding that mission. Their central mission and philosophy drive their decision-making process, and all action stems from this molten core.*

We can see philosophy as our map and mission as our compass or GPS. If you intend to sail a ship from New York to Spain and don't have a map and navigation system, you have much weaker chance of reaching your destination, if any at all. Even if you do get to your destination, there is no doubt that the trip will be much longer and will waste precious resources. It's just more intelligent, efficient, and precise to use a map and navigation system when embarking on a journey from one place to another.

Apple founder Steve Jobs had a clear, well-thought-out philosophy for the vision and mission he had for computers in relation to improving our connection to each other and the world we live in. Once Apple let go of its core philosophy, the company started to tank. It was not until it brought back Steve Jobs and his core philosophy that Apple became one of the world's wealthiest companies. This is a clear-cut modern-day example of how philosophy attached to a mission influences that mission's impact and outcome in the world.

D. D. Palmer discovered chiropractic and wrote his thoughts, ideas, and philosophical concepts in The Chiropractor's Adjustor *in 1910. What is key to understand is that Palmer laid out before us the core and central mission of* chiropractic, which is the location, analysis, and correction of vertebral subluxation with a focus that is nontherapeutic in nature. The core mission must remain the same, or we have something other than chiropractic. What must constantly evolve is the philosophy, science, and art of this mission; otherwise, we have a profession that becomes dogmatic in nature.

B. J. Palmer became the developer of chiropractic, and in his green books volumes 2, 3, 4, 5, and 7, he laid out his vision for the principles on which chiropractic would anchor.

Then, in 1927, R. W. Stephenson came along, and out came a chiropractic textbook that placed many of D. D. Palmer's and B. J. Palmer's principles and concepts into an easily digestible format for teaching. The thirty-three principles gave us a logical, deductive navigation system to understand the why behind this amazing profession we call chiropractic.

I have read the thirty-three principles hundreds of times and have made it my mission that my practices and life are a living testament to these principles in action. Through careful study and application, I believe they can be applied to every and any situation to bring about clarity, success, logic, and understanding in both life and practice.

In this body of work, I asked thirty-three different chiropractors to answer the following four questions in regard to each principle:

1. How do you explain this principle to the public?
2. How does this principle relate to the correction of vertebral subluxation and the practice of chiropractic?
3. Can you give some examples of this principle in action?
4. How does this principle relate to life?

Interwoven between each principle, you will also find practice tips, insights, and quotes to make this book as practical as possible while giving many different opinions and voices. Thank you for participating in this journey with me.

Disclaimer

• • •

Each contribution is the author's own unique interpretation and opinion. The authors, including myself, do not necessarily agree with one another or endorse all the suggestions or insights within this book. Each contributed their own piece of work. It is my hope that 33 brings about scholarly discussion that leads to the evolution of our profession and the advancement of our own lives and practices. I don't believe any one of us has the truth, but all of us working together toward a common vision can uplift and advance chiropractic, leading to greater impact on humanity.

My Journey
Dr. David Serio

• • •

A small body of determined spirits fired by an unquenchable faith in their mission can alter the course of history.

—Mahatma Gandhi

Outstanding people have one thing in common: an absolute sense of mission.

—Zig Ziglar

I feel it is of *value to share a brief version of my journey so the reader understands my* why *for writing this book and the background and context in which it is written.*

I grew up in Fairfield, New Jersey, and was a football player all throughout high school. Most of my teammates and friends would visit chiropractors. They swore by their chiropractors but never could really explain what chiropractic was. They only said it worked wonders for pain. Not having any pain at the time, in my young mind, I saw no reason to go to a chiropractor.

I went off to college and studied marketing. After I graduated, I moved to New York City and worked for AT&T in sales for a few years. One weekend, my friends and I decided to go on a ski trip, and I skied all out all weekend. On Monday, I could not walk and was in severe pain. I thought about my options and decided that it was time to see a chiropractor. At this point, a lot of my coworkers were seeing the company chiropractor and told me he worked miracles with back pain.

My first visit went like this. I walked into this beautiful and very large office space and was given a ton of paperwork to fill out. They took my insurance card and shuffled me off to receive a massage and all types of exams by people who were not the chiropractor. When the chiropractor finally came in, he told me if I didn't see him three times a day for two months, I might never walk again. He proceeded to adjust me and said that my pain would go away within twelve visits. I was very skeptical, and the whole thing seemed set up more as a business than a service to help people.

I can remember this next step as clearly today as the day it happened. I walked out of his office and was right near the Flatiron Building in New York City. It was an amazingly sunny day. People were everywhere, and the sky was crystal blue. I felt this connection to the universe that I had never ever felt in my life. Something profoundly shifted within my being, although I had the same physical pain in my body. At this very moment, I knew I had found my purpose.

Even though my first experience with chiropractic was one of fear, skepticism, and confusion, the adjustment that day shifted my being forever. I will be forever grateful for this chiropractor. Within fifteen days, I had met two other chiropractors through friends. At this point, I switched chiropractors because the first chiropractor was arrested for insurance fraud within seven days of my first visit. In all of my twenty-something years, I had never formally met a chiropractor, and within fifteen days, I knew three. I became friends with one of them, and he told me I should be a chiropractor. I immediately said yes! I quit my job and headed off to Life College where Dr. Sid Williams was president.

My first chiropractor changed my life with an adjustment but clearly did not understand ethical service or the principles of chiropractic. As a result, his practice members never got the full impact of chiropractic, and he ended up on a very dark path. I don't want this scenario to ever happen to another chiropractor or the people he or she serves. We have such a beautiful profession, and the world needs our vision, our principles, and the adjustment of spine and mind now more than ever.

Dr. Sid Williams and Dr. Fred Barge became my first official mentors, and for them, I am forever grateful, because they gave me the fire for my purpose.

While at Life College, I pledged the Delta Sigma Chi fraternity, which brought me deeper into the philosophy of chiropractic. But something inside of me told me there was another angle to our philosophy, a depth that I was missing. About one year into my studies, I heard Arno Burnier and Reggie Gold back-to-back speaking to over 150 students and chiropractors. I was transformed and mystified by the words that so eloquently spiraled off their tongues—the tone, the logic, and the profoundness of their message. I was home.

At the time, Life College was having major issues with accreditation, so I transferred to Sherman College of Straight Chiropractic (as it was called then). The founder and current president was Thom Gelardi. It was here that Thom Gelardi, Reggie Gold, and Arno Burnier became my next three mentors. Soon after, I had the great fortune to be mentored by Joe Strauss, Joe Donofrio (the godfather of Chiropractic), and Donny Epstein.

Once I graduated, I decided that I wanted to see the power of this universal principle in action. What better way to test myself and chiropractic than to move to a foreign country in which I didn't speak the language and where chiropractic was not an established profession? Argentina chose me, and I moved along with another chiropractor just as Argentina was heading into a major depression. Talk about life challenges! Little did I know, but the most challenging yet deeply rewarding years of my journey were about to begin—and continue until this very day…

Throughout the book you will find my contributions in italics.

The most beautiful thing we can experience is the mysterious. It is the source of all true art and science.

—Albert Einstein

PRINCIPLE 1

The Major Premise
Arno Burnier, DC

● ● ●

There is a universal intelligence in all matter, which continually gives to it all its properties and actions, thus maintaining it in existence.

How do I explain this principle to the public?

THIS DEFINITION OF UNIVERSAL INTELLIGENCE is the very foundation of chiropractic, its major premise, from which everything else is deduced. From this general principle, we can deduce all the specifics, down to the cellular and molecular level.

At first, this was just a definition I had to memorize for my class and test on chiropractic philosophy taught by Reginald Gold, DC, while I was at Sherman College of Chiropractic in 1973.

Following numerous repetitions, it began to sink in. I could remember it. I passed my test. Yet it had not taken root in the depth of my being. It had no practical purpose in my life at first.

Then, over time, it hit me in a flash. All matter is infused with universal intelligence. Universal intelligence is omnipresent. It is in every speck of matter, from large objects to the most microscopic particle of matter, to a photon.

We live in a soup of intelligence. We are impregnated, imbued, infiltrated, and bathed in a vast ocean of intelligence.

There is really no place to look for it, for there is no place where it is not.

It is as much present in a church as in a public bathroom or in nature. The entire universe is filled with universal intelligence, also called God, the unified field, the matrix, the explicate order, and the field of all potentiality.

It is said that universal intelligence is a circle, whose center is everywhere and whose circumference is nowhere. This is a great way of referring to the indescribable.

Universal is the cause of all causes. It is source. It is omnipresent, omniscient, and omnipotent. From the great field of "everythingness" or "nothingness" arise all possibilities. *Nothingness* might be a better word to bring to mind the great emptiness from which anything and everything can emerge. *Everythingness* does not confer, in most minds, the infiniteness of endless possibilities.

The term *universal intelligence* might be more accurate than the word *God*; although a rose by any other name is still a rose.

Being raised in the Catholic faith, as a child, I could not come to grip with an omnipresent, omniscient, omnipotent God living somewhere in the universe, keeping track of and tabs on everyone's actions every second of our lives. So as I grew up, I dismissed the whole premise and rejected most of the Catholic doctrine. I embraced the life and message of Christ. I embraced love.

As an adult, when I stumbled into chiropractic philosophy and its major premise of universal intelligence, I felt I could relate and conceptualize in a more accurate way what is inconceivable. I could do that a lot better than believing blindly in some kind of humanlike celestial being called God. In the light of the fact that the word *God* has had so many interpretations, leading to countless wars and unimaginable suffering, *universal intelligence* appears to be a safe term. No one can personify or humanize or put on a pedestal the word *intelligence*.

Would anyone claim that *his or her* universal intelligence is better or greater or different than someone else's universal intelligence? Would anyone fight over whose universal intelligence to follow? Would religious zealots massacre entire indigenous peoples because their universal intelligence is not as universal as theirs? Universal is universal after all.

My experience has been that in sharing the major premise of chiropractic, in teaching about universal intelligence, the faith of religious and spiritual people has deepened. It made their conception and understanding of God more acceptable. They gain a deeper sense of connection with the divinity emanating from the term *God* when connecting to universal intelligence.

It gave them a real understanding that all thoughts, actions, emotions, and deeds are actually connected to all others and known to universal intelligence through the invisible, intangible, incomprehensible, unimaginable, and unfathomable field of intelligence.

How does principle 1 apply to the practice and the adjustment of vertebral subluxation?

From a practical standpoint, since universal intelligence is omnipresent, it permeates, impregnates, and infiltrates every atom, molecule, cell, tissue, organ, and system of our body and being.

That part of universal intelligence that inhabits and flows through a living being, we term *innate intelligence* in chiropractic philosophy. This allows for the distinction between *source*, which is universal intelligence, and semi source, which is innate intelligence. Because, of course, innate intelligence is not the cause or source of everything that exists and will ever exist in the universe. That privilege is left to universal intelligence. It is the only source and cause of everything within a living being.

Just as a drop of ocean water is part of the ocean, innate intelligence is part of universal intelligence. It inherently possesses all the characteristics, properties, and qualities of universal intelligence. Innate intelligence is also omnipresent, omnipotent, and omniscient in living beings. It also possesses the capacity of infinite correlations. This accounts for the myriads of biochemical processes and physiological actions taking place every second of our lives, outside our conscious awareness. How quickly we would fall apart if we had to orchestrate and control such an internal universe. How desperate we would all be to stay alive while sleeping if we had to handle such unimaginable fireworks and computations taking place within the microcosmos of our being.

The realization and knowledge about innate intelligence is empowering and gives people the gift of regaining the authority of their own being.

It gives them knowledge, faith, and trust in the power of their being and body.

Indeed, we are all created from an invisible microscopic dot, the egg. From that minuscule cell, a human being can unfold. This clearly demonstrates that within that original cell reside the power, knowledge, and capacity to create a whole human being. The fertilized egg possesses the knowledge of embryology, dermatology, myology, neurology, cardiology, syndesmology, nephrology, endocrinology, immunology, and osteology to name but a few of the "ologies" that encompasses all the sciences of life.

All principles of physics, chemistry, biology, mechanics, architecture, and any other uncovered sciences and bodies of knowledge already existed in all human beings before any of the *discoverers* of these sciences were ever born.

This realization is both humbling and sobering. We can indeed trust that which created us. Universal intelligence did not abandon us the day we were born. It is alive and well from conception to transition, on the job 24-7, 365 days a year, without ever missing a beat.

The chemistry, biology, immunology, and outcome of trust are a wide departure from that of fear. Trust is actually a real chemical reaction in every single cell of the body. The spectrum of healing that manifests when a person operates in total trust is beyond the average human's wildest imagination. Most of what is required is to drop the barriers of negative expectations.

Innate intelligence utilizes the nervous system as a communication system between the brain and body. The neuro-spinal system is the major pipeline of information, life-force, and chi in the body. It is where the inner net of the body resides. So clearing the neuro-spinal of vertebral subluxation is a positive for human physiology, regardless of age, condition, or symptomatology. We are always better off with a clear channel of communication.

Here is a clear example of principle 1 in action:

Christopher Reeve, the embodiment of Superman, was reduced to a vegetative life due to the interference caused by a broken vertebra in the upper cervical region. His lungs, stomach, kidneys, muscles, and immune system failed to function because of spinal cord compression in the upper neck. His life was shortened by a marked interference between brain and body.

Chiropractic recognizes the paramount importance of clear communication between brain and body. It emphasizes the value of regular checkups and adjustments if needed in order to keep the "garden of our body" supplied with a par level of water, which is life-force in the body.

B. J. Palmer, DC, the developer of chiropractic stated, "Chiropractic adds life to years and years to life" and "The sole purpose of the adjustment is to unify man the spiritual with man the physical." This says it all.

How Does the Major Premise Apply to Life?

The realization of universal intelligence as an omnipresence allows us to accept what has happened and is happening without judgment. It calls us to accept reality for what it is. Embracing what is eradicates unnecessary stress in life. As we have been told countless times, every time we argue with reality, we lose.

There is a valuable practical application of universal intelligence: the possibility of taping, listening to its broadcast by quieting our educated mind. This is best accomplished through meditation, contemplation, or quiet times in nature. This is mostly when the human receiver can tune in and download through inspiration.

Human consciousness is evolving. It may take time to relinquish old ideas and paradigms. Chiropractic philosophy, enunciated by D. D. and B. J. Palmer, might take years to take hold, yet as much as it was put to paper in the early nineteen hundreds, it is as forefront, visionary, and contemporary as ever.

Our Time Has Come

● ● ●

To take in a new idea you must destroy the old, let go of all old opinions, to observe and conceive new thoughts. To learn is but to change your opinion.

—B. J. Palmer

If you want small changes in your life, work on your attitude. But if you want big and primary changes, work on your paradigm.

—Stephen Covey

Craziness is asking people to adapt to cultural customs that create sickness, take us away from our human potential, and create imbalance. Craziness is thinking that sickness care will bring our nations back to health and life. Craziness is thinking that anything that cannot be explained by the mechanistic model of life is unscientific and invalid.

There has never ever been a better time for chiropractic to embrace and be proud of its essence and vitalistic roots. All life and planetary systems are in a crux. There is a great divide. More people are waking up than ever; at the same time, more are asleep.

The world is craving a new philosophy of life on all levels. I believe our principles can be applied to all systems of life, such as health care, the economy, education, politics, and society as well as our individual family systems to create a more harmonious, vital, and sustainable planet.

Our time has come to take this philosophy and make it mainstream. The world needs a new "normal." We have gone so far from the universal principle that for the first time in the history of the human race, people are living fewer years and with less quality than the generation before them.

There has never been a better time to be a chiropractor. We have the chance to assist the planet in a conscious transition and awakening through adjusting spines and minds.

> **A new scientific truth does not triumph by convincing its opponents and making them see the light, but rather because its opponents eventually die, and a new generation grows up that are familiar with it.**
>
> —MAX PLANCK

PRINCIPLE 2

The Chiropractic Meaning of Life
Bill Decken, DC, LCP

• • •

The expression of this intelligence through matter is the chiropractic meaning of life.

Ask a non philosopher, "What do philosophers discuss?" and a likely answer will be "The meaning of life." Ask the same question to a philosopher, and you will rarely get this answer. In the philosophical community, there appears to be a disinterest in this question, and it is likely due to the question's lack of clarity.

Chiropractic is defined in Stephenson's *Chiropractic Text Book* as a philosophy, science, and art of things natural, a system of adjusting the segments of the spinal column by hand only, for the correction of the cause of disease. It is not my intention to discuss this definition in its entirety here, as it does not relate to my topic. I do, however, want to point out that since chiropractic claims to be a philosophy and since the perception by outsiders is that philosophy looks at meaning, then perhaps it was important that the chiropractic founders explain the "meaning of life."

It is interesting to note that chiropractic principles essentially begin with the meaning of life and the discussion of it is carried all the way through to principle 33. No place in the principles is health discussed. Instead, what Stephenson described as a deductive science of life commences with a general statement about all matter and concludes with a very specific statement about a subluxation interfering with expression in living (vertebrate) matter.

When I was young boy playing baseball, the coach could frequently be heard yelling at us to "show some life." He wanted us to look alive and not like a bump on a log. Life, in this case, meant motion, activity, an appearance that we were "in the game."

Growing up, when we were not feeling too great or were downright sick, my mother would say we looked "like death warmed over." Well, let's think about that. When we are under the weather, not feeling too well, don't we look different? Don't we look like our energy levels are down? Is there not a visible change in our countenance? My mom was not a trained scientist, but she sure seems to have hit the vibrational energy concept in science exactly right. She noticed that we were vibrating on a different level, and sure enough, death and life have different vibrations, different expressions.

So what makes matter vibrate? Science tells us that all matter has vibrations. The human body consists of matter, as does the kitchen table. Both are made of atoms, and all atoms are vibrating at some level. There is a universal intelligence expressed in the molecular structure of the material the table is made from, and there is also educated intelligence expressed in the design and function of the table. Innate intelligence is expressed in the human being sitting at the table. Three types of intelligence are all being expressed in matter, and yet we only have "control" over one of them, the educated intelligence. We see expression of all three forms of intelligence by way of the efficiency, organization, and purposefulness with which the matter functions.

The previous principle (1) started with the assumption that matter is organized by a universal intelligence, and in that organization, we see properties and actions being expressed. It will, therefore, make perfect sense later on when we concern ourselves with the expression of intelligence in living matter, the people getting checked in our offices.

So, in chiropractic, the meaning of life is the expression of intelligence through matter. Young ballplayers give meaning to the game by expressing the actions of a ballplayer. The kitchen table takes on the meaning it was intended to have, whether that be a place for us to sit comfortably while dining or having great family interaction. Michelangelo's *David* gets its meaning from the properties of the marble from which it was derived. Similarly, young children may express the actions and properties of robust health one day and look like death warmed over the next. In both cases, the children are expressing the purposefulness of their physiological functions. In both cases, their body is working efficiently and in an organized fashion to adapt to the situation at hand. These are all examples of different types of matter expressing different types of intelligence. They all have a measure of life.

When chiropractors develop a continuing education program for their practice members, they mostly focus on the expression of innate and educated intelligence in the matter of the person's body. In addition, this principle, 2, will be crucial in understanding the simplicity and logic of several later principles that are also used frequently in educating folks about chiropractic.

For instance, the muscles (matter) of an active, athletic person palpate much differently than those of a couch potato. In both cases, educated intelligence is being expressed because it was educated intelligence that made the lifestyle choice. A similar comparison could be made between a desk job and manual labor or between various nutritional regimens.

Regardless of which person we are palpating, we will be able to palpate the working muscles that move the vertebrae. We will also be able to measure the heat patterns along the spine as well as the electrical activity of the paraspinal muscles. These are all expressions of the innate intelligence of the body.

As the person moves forward with regular chiropractic care, the correction of subluxations will allow for the better expression of the innate intelligence of the body. This will be made evident by differences in the matter of the body as the body begins to give evidence of a more efficient, organized, and purposeful expression of life. We will note changes in palpation, thermography, and myography, to name just a few.

There is a difference between a fast-moving stream in the woods, with an aura of vibrancy, and one that is meandering and dying. Both are expressing life but at different levels. When subluxation is present, the nerve traffic is not moving, like a dying stream. When the nerve system is clear of interference, it is like a fast-moving stream, full of energy, power, and life.

Do you see properties and actions in the world around you? Does your practice member see, hear, smell, taste, or feel anything about his or her body? It is intelligence being expressed. It has meaning. Seek to understand it.

Practice Pre-Game

● ● ●

Be a yardstick of quality. Some people aren't used to
an environment where excellence is expected.

—Steve Jobs

The two most important days of your life are the
day you were born and the day you find out why.

—Mark Twain

The practice of chiropractic is *not a mechanistic venture. The practice of chiropractic is a reflection of its principles in action. The practice takes on a living morphic field of its own. I often compare the practice to human life. The first nine months before you open your practice, your practice is like a baby growing in the womb. You are preparing for the practice to be born.*

Arno Burnier always told me to first see the adjustment in my mind's eye. Visualization is essential for creating your dream practice. But in order to do this, you must answer some essential questions from a place of self-awareness.

Translated to Action

What is your why? *What is the reason you are a chiropractor? What drives you to awake each day and take action?*

Have you defined your purpose? Mission? Vision? Have you mapped out your five highest values in life and as a chiropractor? Do you have clear objectives for your health, practice, family, economics, and professional career?

Before you can even think about embarking on something as serious as opening a chiropractic practice, I would suggest you get your personal stuff in order and have clearly defined all of the above in detail and with total clarity.

Two of my highest values as a chiropractor are the following:

1. *To clear vertebral subluxations from as many people as humanly possible so they can express life more fully at every level*
2. *To assist people in living with a deeper connection to the universal principle and their inner intelligence through sharing the thirty-three principles and the philosophy of chiropractic*

Every single aspect and detail of the physical space to the systems I developed has complete integration and alignment with the 33 principles and my highest life and chiropractic values. I visualized, felt, and experienced the entire experience of my practice from the first phone call to my clients' visits thirty years down the line. I asked myself at least two hundred questions in regard to my practice before ever seeing one person.

What techniques would I use? Would I use instrumentation? Would I check people fully clothed or skin on skin? If I was to gown people, how could I do this in a high-volume setting? What type of tables would I purchase? What type of music would I play? Would there be colors on the wall? How did I want my checking rooms set up for maximum efficiency? What would my assistant be like? Would I have a children's area, and what would it look like? What information would I have out for people to take home? What would my educational program consist of? How would people start care in my practice? What type of people did I want to attract? Since I wanted to serve as many people as possible, what price point would be congruent with this thinking? The list went on and on until every single minor and major detail felt right within me.

What is important to understand is that the "dream" practice does not have to be what you manifest on day 1. You can take each piece of a practice and make improvements little by little, depending on your financial situation. The important step is to know exactly what you want, what is fully aligned with your heart, and the steps you need to take to get there.

Once you have all the basis set you are ready for your practice to be "born". This is where the "triune of practice" must come into full fruition. Intelligence-You must practice in an efficient and intelligent manner using a system that has a purpose to every single detail. Force-If you want to grow a practice you must put force or energy into it understanding the universal principle that energy output will equal a specific outcome. Quite simply, the more energy you put into the practice both internally and externally the bigger and faster it will grow. Matter-Your practice should be physically clean, professional, stylish and the level of mastery to your physical craft will have a major impact on how deeply you effect lives. The Triune of your practice will either move towards growth or away from growth and it all depends upon YOU!

An unexamined life is not worth living.

—SOCRATES

PRINCIPLE 3

The Union of Intelligence and Matter
Gilles A. LaMarche, DC

● ● ●

Life is necessarily the union of intelligence and matter.

A PRINCIPLE IS DEFINED AS a fundamental truth or proposition that serves as the foundation for a system of belief or behavior or for a chain of reasoning. The thirty-three principles of chiropractic are exactly that, a series of fundamental truths.

Principle 3 is the union of intelligence and matter—*life is necessarily the union of intelligence and matter*. For many, this may sound somewhat abstract, but once you understand, you come to realize how simple and yet profound this principle—and all thirty-three—really is. So what does "union of intelligence and matter" really mean? Did you ever stop to wonder how everything in the universe works? How your mind and body work? How two cells can come together and in forty weeks create some forty billon cells, ten toes and ten fingers, beautiful eyes, a smile, an ability to feed, a nervous system that will control all functions, including respiration, digestion, elimination, and sexual reproduction later in life, and so much more? Some of you may have, and others may not yet have done so. Let's consider it together right now. If you reread principle 1, you know "there is a universal intelligence in all matter..." What does that mean to you? To me, it means that there is a power that governs everything that happens in our beautiful universe, and this same power governs you. So imagine if you will this intelligence, this software program being operated by the world's most gigantic computer, the universe's greatest mind.

Everything that happens around you—the sun rising, the clouds forming, rivers flowing, birds singing, grass and flowers growing—*everything* is governed by this intelligence we call universal intelligence. And now imagine that this same intelligence is put into you and called innate intelligence. Every living person has innate intelligence, or he or she wouldn't be living. Every organic function—your heart beating, your lungs breathing, your stomach digesting, your kidneys filtering, your liver ridding your body of toxins, your ability to think, your willingness to smile, your eyes capturing images being interpreted by your brain, your ears hearing, your nose smelling—is proof positive that this intelligence exists inside of you. The vast majority of people do not realize this and go about their lives unconscious of this superb power. The only difference between someone living and someone dead is that innate intelligence animates the living being. Innate intelligence is the silent partner, unobservable and unknown, yet as real as life. Innate intelligence is the wholesome and reliable knowledge of all things and functions that take place without you even knowing. When innate intelligence is unified to your body (matter), you are living, and when innate intelligence leaves your body, you are not. That's why we say that *life is necessarily the union of intelligence and matter.*

Chiropractic's goal is to maximize the expression of your perfection within, allowing your innate intelligence to be fully expressed throughout your life. We recognize that you, your mind and body, like all other organic systems in the universe, are self-developing, self-maintaining, and self-healing and that these systems work best when they are free of interference. Your nervous system is responsible for orchestrating the internal and external dialogue of your body necessary for life to be fully expressed. We also recognize that there are three interferences to proper nervous system function—physical trauma, environmental toxins, and emotional stress. Your body's inability to adapt to these stresses leads to subluxations that invariably can create a spiraling decline in your health expression. This creates decreased expression of innate intelligence within your body, commonly explained as a disconnection of innate intelligence to matter. Therefore, our purpose is to correct these interferences, via a chiropractic adjustment, allowing you to express your innate potential and live an extraordinary life. Yes, the role of your chiropractor is to detect, analyze, and correct your subluxations and guide you to reduce the interferences that lead to subluxation and decreased quality of life. The longer you are subluxated, the lower your quality of life, even though you may not know it, even though you may not feel it. Pain is the body's way of telling you that something is wrong; however, in many instances, pain is the last thing to show up. Some people have had dysfunction for years before pain and tissue or organ breakdown occur. You certainly know of someone who was told by a physician, after a physical exam, that all looked good and that he or she was healthy. Yet, a short while after, this person had a serious health crisis or may have even died of a massive heart attack or other issue. I ask you this question: "Was that person healthy, or did he or she simply appear to be healthy?" Is it possible that the person had serious subluxations shutting off the flow of innate intelligence to the body, and over time, the systems simply failed? I would venture to say that the answer to these questions is "yes." There was *disunion of intelligence and matter*, instead of *union of intelligence and matter*, and life, as we know it, ended.

Why, for example, does an individual live the first four or five decades of his or her life appearing completely healthy and all of a sudden die of a massive heart attack? Why does a virus or bacteria create sniffles in one child and a serious disease in a sibling? Is it not logical to assume that if an individual is born completely normal with all systems functioning to the optimum that this individual is healthy and should in fact live a long life and die healthy? Would it not be normal to recognize that death is nothing more than part of the great master plan of life? If science today tells us that the human body is created to last 120 to 150 years, why then is this not the case?

D. D. Palmer, the discoverer of chiropractic, said this: "I desired to know why one person was ailing and his associate, eating at the same table, working at the same shop…was not. Why? What difference was there in the two persons that caused one to have disease while his partner escaped? Why?"

When there is a disconnection between innate intelligence and your body (matter), you cannot and will not be healthy; it's that simple. Will knowing this critical information change how you view health? Will it change how you choose to maintain your health? Will you make better decisions beginning today for both yourself and your family?

Knowing that *life is necessarily the union of intelligence and matter* and that subluxations lead to the *disunion of intelligence and matter*, which leads to decreased quality of life and premature death, should be enough to get you to be regularly checked by your chiropractor and adjusted when necessary, don't you think? I certainly hope you said a very loud *yes*!

Tonality

• • •

Life is the expression of tone. In that sentence
is the basic principle of chiropractic.

—D. D. Palmer

If you want to find the secrets of the universe, think
in terms of energy, frequency and vibration.

—Nikola Tesla

According to leading sales expert *Jordan Belfort, also known as the Wolf of Wall Street, tone and energy are almost 85 percent or more of what inspires people to buy from you. The science of sales shows that our words have meaning but are much less of a factor than we think in any type of sales transaction. Your tone in practice must be inspiring, exuding confidence and clarity, and infused with love if you are going to attract the masses of people to choose chiropractic in your practice.*

Some people are natural tonality masters, and some work very, very hard on this aspect of their being. Jordan Belfort and the masters of NLP agree that anyone can learn techniques to master tonality. Tesla and D. D. Palmer stated very clearly that tonality is one of the keys and secrets to life. You can be the best analyzer and adjustor of vertebral subluxation and have the best office and systems, but if your tone is less than optimal, you will have a hard time building your dream practice! Do whatever you need to do to become a master at tonality, and watch your practice and life take on a whole different meaning.

One of the most powerful things about moving to a country in which I did not speak a word of the language is that I had to become a master of tonality in order to communicate. This means not only mastering my tonality but also understanding the tonality of listening. What I have personally learned and experienced in this situation is that typically people's words don't match their tonality, so the truth of what they're saying can be felt and not heard in their words. If you become a master at picking up tonality, you will be able to read the real truth and energy behind what people are saying. This brings a power to communication beyond what you can imagine.

This understanding enables you to tap into people's hearts and minds on a level that goes so far beyond verbal communication. As you start to master tonality, you will become a much more powerful person in all aspects of your life and practice. You will attract with ease as if you were the world's most powerful magnet, and practice becomes stress-free. Any Chiropractor who has made major impact in his or her community, practice, or our profession has understood and transmitted tonality on some level of mastery.

Change your tone, change your life.

—DAVID SERIO, DC

PRINCIPLE 4

The Triune of Life
Mark Romano, DC

● ● ●

Life is a triunity having three necessary united factors, namely, intelligence, force, and matter.

THIS PRINCIPLE IS AN EASY idea to observe but a challenging one to measure. We can use logic with the public when we observe the organization of matter. Using the human body, for example, it is obvious to see that the body is highly organized in its structure and function. Logic would tell us that there cannot be organization without intelligence. The human body and its literally countless physiological functions demonstrate incredible organization and adaptive qualities. The intelligence that controls these functions resides within the body (known in chiropractic as innate intelligence), and it is expressed through force.

The force created by innate intelligence is designed to adapt matter for its survival, existence, and progress. Matter depends on this force for coordination and adaption to occur. How humbling it is that two of the three components of this principle are metaphysical and beyond measure. Working with the human body is humbling for any profession because the body is a synergistic organism. It is simply greater than the sum of its parts. Having this understanding is vital to our ability to maximize our life experience and serve others, in this case, through chiropractic. Within the body, we have two intelligences, innate (or inborn) and educated. We do our best to measure them, but both fall short of being measured. Innate intelligence is inborn. The body has 100 percent knowledge of how to coordinate all body functions, and it stays at this 100 percent ability until we die. Educated intelligence is acquired through life. It starts at zero, and we begin to learn from birth. Many scientists believe that this intelligence peaks at a certain age and then begins a decline in later years of life. Educated intelligence is measured often in school through tests, boards, and so on. And as we have seen repeatedly, people can score poorly on tests in school and do amazing and accomplish things at an incredibly high intellectual level in their chosen career.

Knowing intelligence is challenging to measure opens us up to humble observation of innate intelligence within the matter it resides. This brings us to how principle 4 relates to the essence of chiropractic. As we stated, innate intelligence is always 100 percent and is always aware of every need of the matter in which it resides. Innate intelligence creates force that is necessary to adapt and coordinate the function of matter. The force created by innate intelligence can be interfered with, therefore creating incoordination in matter. This puts matter in a state of *dis*-ease, being less than at ease. One of the ways innate intelligence can be interfered with is the chiropractic entity called a vertebral subluxation. A vertebral subluxation is a condition of a vertebra that has lost its proper juxtaposition with the one above, the one below, or both, to an extent less than a luxation, which impinges nerves and interferes with the transmission of mental impulses. This is one of the most powerful discoveries perhaps in the history of humankind. It simply states that a bone in our spine can misalign and produce nerve interference of some kind and interfere with the force created by innate intelligence (at this point, a mental impulse), thus causing the body to function at less than 100 percent. This is *powerful*! Simply stated, the body will never reach its fullest potential so long as vertebral subluxations are present. What a powerful purpose and impact chiropractors have on the whole human race!

Vertebral subluxations occur when the external invasionary forces overcome the internal resistive force. This can happen any day or every day. Vertebral subluxations have no symptomatic or clinical presentation because the majority of body function occurs beyond our human awareness. Therefore, the only way anyone can know if a vertebral subluxation is present in the spine is to see a chiropractor to have the spinal analyzed. Vertebral subluxations destroy lives. The correction of vertebral subluxations on a regular basis allows mental impulse to be expressed, and people's bodies can adapt more fully, thus improving quality of life in every way imaginable.

Examples of this principle are everywhere—in living matter and in nonliving matter. A rock demonstrates intelligent design in its qualities and characteristics. The rock was created by an intelligence (universal intelligence). Universal intelligence uses force to express itself through the matter of the rock. It organizes the rock, gives it predictable qualities, and maintains its existence. The organization can be observed in the color of the rock and physical qualities, such as melting point, boiling point, and molecular bonds.

Examples of this principle are obvious in all living matter. Observation tells us so much. In observing humans, we see coordinated function and adaption to the internal and external environments in a person we would call healthy. We see the presence of intelligence in matter because matter is very highly organized in humans, and there cannot be organization without intelligence. We also see this principle, or lack thereof, in someone we would call sick, unhealthy, or lacking health. The matter is not fully adapting, and there are physiological demonstrations that would support lack of adaption. This can be deceiving at times for many reasons. First, some symptoms that seem nonadaptive could actually be highly adaptive. One example is vomiting. A person may vomit because his or her body is not adapting to its fullest potential *or* because it is adapting very well and is getting rid of something poisonous or dangerous to body function. At times, it can be impossible to differentiate the two possibilities. Another possible occurrence is the body is not adapting and functioning at its fullest potential, perhaps because of vertebral subluxations or another issue, but the lack of adaption is not observable. This is another reason why humility helps us in working with the human body.

This principle relates to life in many powerful ways. It defines life in both its physical and metaphysical components. This principle exploits the absolute necessity of humility when working with the human body. This principle truly shows just how much ahead of their time our forebears were in their thinking and commitment to excellence, chiropractic, and humankind. As we have stated, intelligence is an abstract. Force created by intelligence is an abstract. Both are beyond measure, but both can be observed through the observation of matter. Life, the essence of all living and nonliving things, expresses organization, not chaos. Organization simply cannot live without intelligence. The chiropractic meaning of life is the expression of this intelligence through matter by force. Observation with logic is a powerful tool. There is so much growth and understanding yet to be accomplished in chiropractic. Our forebears started us on a powerful journey. We do not need to know everything or see everything. We just need to see the next step. And with each step, our view and knowledge improve, my friends!

KISS

• • •

Simplicity is the ultimate sophistication.

—LEONARDO DA VINCI

Simplicity and repose are qualities that measure the true value of any work of art.

—FRANK LLOYD WRIGHT

KISS. KEEP IT SIMPLE, STUPID.

All spiritual teachings at some point teach the power of simplicity.

When you are designing your practice, I urge you to ask yourself this question. Is this procedure, detail, system or form of communication as simple as it can be? If the answer is yes, leave it alone. If not, simplify. People want simplicity. They crave simplicity. In today's world, they don't want more complexity. They crave simplicity, love, connection, touch, wisdom, and inspiration—all things we can easily create in our practices that stem from simplicity.

If you think about the most powerful things we can do for our lives and health, they are all very simple. A chiropractic adjustment is a very simple thing to give and receive, yet it transforms our being in an instant. Walking is simple to do and has a profound impact on our health. Eating simply is much better than making our diet complex. Meditation is so simple it can be done anywhere, at any time, and yet it has a profound physiological impact. A smile is a simple thing to give and receive, yet it profoundly shifts the physiology of the giver and receiver. The list goes on and on.

Universal law is simple. Its application is simple. The impact is infinite.

This is where the real power of chiropractic lies. It is a simple philosophy with a simple application, yet it has profound effects on every aspect of the human experience. All we really need is our heart, head, and hands to perform our craft and serve people with the gift of chiropractic. As the world becomes more and more complex, simplicity is quickly becoming the new model of conscious living.

> **To me the extraordinary aspect of martial arts lies in its simplicity. The easy way is also the right way, and martial arts is nothing at all special. The closer to the true way of martial arts, the less wastage of expression there is.**
>
> **—Bruce Lee**

PRINCIPLE 5

The Perfection of the Triune
Stamatis Tsamoutalidis

● ● ●

In order to have 100 percent life, there must be 100 percent intelligence, 100 percent force, and 100 percent matter.

1. How do you explain this principle to the public?
THERE ARE A FEW CHIROPRACTIC principles that can stand alone in their understanding (e.g., principles 6 and 17). For me, principle 5 is much more thoroughly understood when you have access to the other thirty-two principles as well. There are words in this principle that have not been properly defined. (For example, what is force? What is its function? And so on.) So, it takes having access to all the other principles for this one to be best understood.

How much detail you go into on this with the public will be determined by how much they want to learn and how capable they are of learning. But before the chiropractor can explain this principle to the public, it is important for him or her to fully understand this principle.

Let's break it down.

Life is an absolute. When we are talking about universal life (organic or inorganic), it is always 100 percent. The expression of (universal) intelligence through matter is the chiropractic meaning of life (principle 2). If matter did not express intelligence, it would be dead; it would not even exist.

The triune of life requires intelligence, force, and matter (principle 4). The three factors of the triune are inseparable. For there to be 100 percent life, the perfection of the triune must be maintained; they cannot be separated.

Intelligence is infinite and always 100 percent perfect. In a living thing (human body), the intelligence is innate intelligence (principle 20). It is always 100 percent (principle 22), and its mission is to actively organize the materials of the body (principle 21). The function of intelligence is to create force (principle 8) and adapt universal forces and matter for use in the body so that all parts will have coordinated action for mutual benefit (principle 23).

The force created by intelligence is always 100 percent (principle 9). Perfect intelligence cannot create force that is less than perfect. The job of force is to unite intelligence and matter (principle 10). Force transfers intelligence to matter perfectly.

The function of matter is to express force (principle 13). Since all life has motion, there is universal life in all matter (principle 14). Matter is always perfect in the moment.

In a human body, our philosophy teaches us that 100 percent innate intelligence creates 100 percent force. The force is conducted over the nervous system (principle 28), which is matter. If there is a breakdown of the triune, it must be with the matter. Matter is capable of being less than 100 percent in two situations. Both entail the limitations of matter (principle 24).

1. Specifically, with nerve tissue, the matter may not be able to carry the mental impulses to the body parts because of a vertebral subluxation.
2. Even if the body part can receive the mental impulses, it may be so damaged because of trauma, genetic defect, or even absence that it cannot do anything with it.

Now this may seem like it contradicts the principle, but it can be explained in two ways.

1. A body that may be diseased or not expressing 100 percent innate life is still expressing universal life. Remember that this principle ultimately deals with universal life.
2. In a human body, if an organ or body part is removed and there are no vertebral subluxations present, the body can still be a 100 percent expression of the triune. However, compared to what the human body could have been, it is another story since all body parts are necessary for the best ability to adapt in life. Any limitations in the structure of matter reflect an imperfect organization or arrangement of the matter. It, therefore, follows that any imperfection in the expression of intelligence is due to a limitation of matter.

Wrapping all this up, life is 100 percent (whether it is universal or innate). We use our senses to determine that matter exists. Whether it is inorganic (e.g., a rock) or organic (e.g., the human body), the matter exists at 100 percent. At the atomic and subatomic levels, all matter has motion. Force provides that motion in matter. The force is 100 percent because it is created by an intelligence that is 100 percent. When intelligence, force, and matter are 100 percent, so is life.

2. How does this principle apply to the practice of chiropractic and the correction of vertebral subluxation?

Our chiropractic philosophy recognizes the perfection of intelligence and force. Chiropractors try to create an unbroken connection between the three components of the triune. The chiropractic objective is to correct vertebral subluxations to allow the force created by innate intelligence to be better expressed.

As chiropractors, we work with the physical matter of the body. Universal forces can damage the body (principle 26). External invasive forces (physical, chemical, and emotional stress) can overcome the body's internal resistive forces, causing vertebral subluxations. This results in the body (matter), specifically nerve tissue, not being able to carry mental impulses properly.

Our objective is to find and assist in the correction of vertebral subluxations. By restoring normal alignment and function in the spine, we remove interference to the transmission of the forces caused by vertebral subluxations in the matter of the body (specifically nerve tissue). This better allows the force created by the innate intelligence of the body to do what it is created to do. This results in restoration of normal body function.

We hope the matter can then have a better opportunity to do what it needs to do within the limitations of time and matter. However, anything that occurs afterward is an incidental effect.

Also, we recognize that there are many other things that can damage the body and make it function abnormally. Sometimes the damage and abnormal function will be permanent. Poor nutrition, exposure to toxins, lack of movement or exercise, removal of body parts, and so on are just some examples. These issues fall beyond the scope of chiropractic and are best addressed by other professions that specialize in those things.

3. Can you give some examples of this principle in action?

In an ideal situation, we have a fully healthy and unsubluxated person. All body parts are healthy and functioning normally—100 percent matter. There is no interference to the mental impulses generated by innate intelligence—100 percent force. Therefore, the innate intelligence can be expressed perfectly in the body—100 percent intelligence. This is the perfect example of 100 percent life due to 100 percent intelligence, 100 percent force, and 100 percent matter.

Now let's look at a body that has a diseased organ—let's use the kidney as an example. Let's assume the person is under regular chiropractic care and subluxation-free. The (innate) intelligence of the body is 100 percent, and the force is 100 percent, since the person is unsubluxated. The matter that exists will not possess 100 percent normal function (or 100 percent innate life), in that the organ is not 100 percent healthy and functioning like it should. However, the diseased kidney is still expressing universal life in that it exists and in whatever percentage of innate life it can still produce.

Lastly, in this same scenario of a person with a diseased kidney, let's assume the person was not under chiropractic care and was subluxated. The person would still have all the limitations of matter in the previous paragraph. However, he or she would also be dealing with a body that is lacking the proper supply of mental impulses because of a vertebral subluxation. The innate intelligence of the body is 100 percent, the force created by intelligence is 100 percent, but its transmission over the matter (nerve tissue) is interfered with, and the body, as a result, is in a state of dis-ease (incoordination).

4. How does this principle apply to life?

Those of us who understand the importance of chiropractic care will make sure that we, our families, and the people we serve are as subluxation free as possible. This will help to make sure that the 100 percent intelligence and 100 percent force will, we hope, be expressed at 100 percent as much as possible through our bodies (matter).

We also recognize that there are things outside of chiropractic that can contribute to keeping the matter that our bodies are composed of working as best as it can—things like proper nutrition, exercise, and proper rest. We also know that we should avoid as many things that are harmful to our bodies as we can. If we are interested in pursuing those things, we should consult and learn from experts in those areas. Our objective in practice is limited to helping maintain 100 percent life by correcting vertebral subluxations.

Appreciation and Attraction
Richelle Knowles, DC, and Daniel Knowles, DC

● ● ●

As we express our gratitude, we must never forget that the highest appreciation is not to utter words but to live by them.

—John F. Kennedy

Appreciation is the highest form of prayer, for it acknowledges the presence of good wherever you shine the light of your thankful thoughts.

—Alan Cohen

Unfortunately, many people are misled to believe that practice growth is solely the effect of their procedures, their team, their location, their paint color, their posters, and their technique. The reality is that, while all of those things are important, they are not the most important thing. The most important part of your practice is —your practice is not about you.

Once people really get that under their skin, they realize that there's so much more to serving more people on a higher level than all of those things. It will also drive them to better all those aspects of their office that we mentioned because they realize that the real effect that they're looking for is changing people's lives for the better. Until they truly get that under their skin, their practice will be about them. And it will not reach the heights that is possible to reach.

Understand that the reason of any business enterprise is to serve its customers and put its customers' or clients' needs first. When you do that and get obsessed with practice member success, then you realize you have bettered everything about you, not for you, but so that you can better the quality of care that your office delivers.

Furthermore, you realize that rather than blaming your team, your procedures, or your situation for a lack of success, you realize that the success of your practice depends upon you, that you create a field like a vacuum through your office to attract people from everywhere. Building a practice on attraction and appreciation becomes the first order of business.

A hallmark of every aspect of our practice, for decades, has been to have various appreciation programs for our practice members to show how much we love them.

Show your appreciation of them for spending their hard-earned money and their valuable time to travel to your office and receive care. They deserve your best, your presence, your gratitude, and your appreciation, and you must consistently find ways to show that to them. Exceptional service is vital not only to the practice survival but also to the practice thriving.

Commonly, practitioners think that people discontinue care because of financial and time constraints. Those may be the things that people say and that are valid on the surface. The truth is that those become bigger when the value and appreciation people are getting out of visiting the practitioner's office decreases. And for that reason, their priorities shift. The real reason people discontinue with services is feeling taken for granted or not appreciated enough. The more engaged, present, and appreciative the practitioner is with the practice member, the more the person gets out of care.

Your greatest marketing tool is your heart. Grow your heart, grow your love, and grow your appreciation for those you serve first and foremost and above all your other efforts. Then the how of everything else that fits in with your heart-set and mind-set will come to the surface. Yielding the ultimate result that you truly are looking for, which is more people, on more tables, more often.

> **Being told you're appreciated is one of the simplest and most uplifting things you can hear.**
>
> —Author Unknown

PRINCIPLE 6

The Principle of Time
Joe Donofrio, DC, and Mark Romano, DC

● ● ●

There is no process that does not require time.

The relevance of time in our country seems to be the lack of it. We, in the United States, seem to try to fit as much activity as possible into each of our days, seven days a week. Most of us simply run out of time to finish all of our desired activities. It seems we are so busy trying to get things done that we forget to live, enjoy, and invest in our life, and the consequences can be very negative and disempowering. Our culture seems to get so focused on getting things done as quickly as possible that this principle is a vital reminder of the importance of the process within the parameters of time. Our lives are determined by our habits. Our habits are the daily and weekly activities we do over time. Our habits shape our lives over years of repetition. In order to change the quality of our lives, we must change the process of our habits and sustain them through time. This is vital to the public understanding and receiving the full benefit of what chiropractic truly has to offer. Vertebral subluxations occur perhaps daily in all human beings. They occur because of the limitation of matter in which innate intelligence's internal forces are overcome by external universal forces, and the vertebrae (matter) misalign, occluding foramen, impinging nerves, and interfering with the transmission of mental impulse. Let alone, vertebral subluxations produce damage daily, a process through time that causes the body to build damage and disease, keeping one further and further from one's fullest potential. Now, when people become members of our practice, they begin the powerful process of making chiropractic a weekly habit. Through this habit, over years (time), their bodies live less with vertebral subluxations and experience a fuller expression of life (innate intelligence). The importance of this habit cannot be overemphasized. We cannot predict how the body will function better, but logic tells us that the body will be stronger in every way with chiropractic as a weekly habit (process) over time. This makes chiropractic a powerful investment with literally no downside.

The awareness of this principle benefits both the chiropractor and the practice member. It benefits the chiropractor by keeping chiropractic in the non-crisis, non-therapeutic model. The practice member knowing that chiropractic is a process and the chiropractor does not make the adjustment but rather is simply a part of the process allows the chiropractor never to be in a crisis mind-set and always to be specific and gentle in his or her analysis and facilitation of the adjustment.

The practice member benefits by knowing on the front end that chiropractic is a habit and the correction of the vertebral subluxation is a process. It takes time to earn the body's trust and figure out vertebral subluxation patterns. Knowing this, the member can experience the full benefit of chiropractic by making it a routine habit in his or her life.

The quality of our lives is the result of every choice we have made. Our choices become habits, and our habits make the life we lead. We can observe this principle in every facet of our lives, from the quality of our health and strength to our career and relationships. This is powerful because it puts us in control of our life and allows us to break free from the mentality of being a victim or helpless. When we observe people living lives of abundance, health, or financial success, it is easy to see that their lifestyle is not the result of one moment in time or one event in their lives. But rather, it was a process of habit, focus, and action of time that ultimately brought to them life they are living. This principle is also evident on the negative side as well. Those living in a state of depression, dis-ease, poverty, and dissatisfaction with their lives have habits that keep them in the very place they claim to despise. It is powerful knowing that humans have the ability to be self-aware. We can radically change our lives by changing our focus, thoughts, decisions, and habits. The process over time is an empowering concept to living the quality of life we as humans are capable of. Human potential has amazing and unlimited possibilities. We all have limits to our potential. We have yet, as humans, to fully realize what those limits might be. This is so very exciting and empowering as to how far-reaching chiropractic can truly be to humanity.

At first blush, this simplistic statement seems barely worth stating, seeming to be an observation of the obvious requirements of time. However, with thought and, ironically, some time, I came to realize that it was far more about process than it was about time. I have long felt that most chiropractors gloss over the need for time in the process of creation and correction of the vertebral subluxation. Most of us speak on the creation of vertebral subluxation as if it occurs something like the turning off a light switch. We lift something, and a back "goes out"; we sneeze, and "something pops out"; or we step off a curb wrong and get a sudden back spasm or pain. I could go on, but you get the idea. Thus, while it is true that a small number of vertebral subluxations do result from extreme trauma like falling off a roof or being hit by a car, the vast majority are the result of small, even imperceptible, trauma to the soft tissues responsible for maintaining vertebral mobility and position over time. Over time, such trauma creates a small weakness, perhaps in a ligament, and innate intelligence begins a process of healing it with less functional fibrous tissues; this is followed by another and perhaps another similar happening, creating a small weakness in a para-spinal tissue, which is now ripe for a final trauma that may result in some insult to the nervous tissue. Now, finally, after months and years, the vertebral subluxation is beginning to develop into a vertebral subluxation in its full definition and sense. It is a process that requires time, as Stephenson meant in principle 6. The vertebral subluxation is now in full bloom, complete with nerve-impulse interference and dis-ease (notice the hyphen). At this juncture, in walks the chiropractor, who, with his or her analysis, determines the presences and character of the vertebral subluxation. And so begins the next *time*-consuming process, the correction.

In most cases, because a chiropractor is rarely the first professional consulted, the soft tissues around the vertebral subluxation have chronically altered their function and position in innate's attempt to adapt, thus, requiring what I call a "readaption" period before correction can be achieved. Again, this is a process that requires time, perhaps weeks, months, or years. But the correction must become reality if the organism is to ever have any hope of "ease."

It seems to me that the chiropractic profession needs to eliminate its all-too-frequent references to "throwing the switch" and "turning on life" and the like if we are to engender in our members or patients truly honest and reasonable expectations for our care. The understanding of this time process lies at the very heart of the need for lifetime spinal checks, rather than occasional symptomatic care.

Adding Value through Education and Communication

• • •

It is only in your thriving that you have
anything to offer anyone.

—Esther Hicks

People's commitment to your practice will always be
equal to or below your level of commitment to them.

—David Serio, DC

Are new people important? Of course they are! We want to help as many new people as possible, but very often, 90 percent of our focus is on finding new people rather than keeping the ones we have.

I see the practice as an above-down-inside-out venture, just as health and life comes from above-down-inside-out. Thus every detail and system we put in place should have an above-down-inside-out objective.

As I have worked with many chiropractors, it has been my experience that in general people tend to blame everything outside of themselves as to why their practice is not thriving—the economy, holidays, people don't get it in their culture, this time of year people don't start new things, people don't really have time to bring their kids, people are very closed minded in their city, and so on…the list never ends. Outside-in-below-up thinking takes all of the responsibility off you, when in reality, your life is 100 percent your responsibility. Sustainable success is an above-down-inside-out process.

Practical Action

Jordan Belfort, the Wolf of Wall Street, says people will judge you in an instant on three things.

1. Are you inspired?
2. Are you sharp as a tack?
3. Do you have something that will empower them?

You are only as good as your last visit. So number one, you must have these three qualities each and every visit. You want to keep people? Then you must inspire them with your enthusiasm for serving them chiropractic, educating them, and empowering them each and every visit. Your communication must be powerful, direct, and clear.

Develop on ongoing education program. In our practice, we approach people on the first visit as if they will stay with us for life.

First Visit

We have a forty-five-minute talk, introducing them to key concepts of chiropractic and our practice.

This is the visit in which we are dressed to impress. We share our hearts and passion and have a talk that is logical, clear, and concise and has tons of visuals and examples. We share information that is empowering in nature rather than fear driven.

Twenty-Five-Visit Educational Program

We have twenty-five professionally designed educational pieces explaining key principles and concepts that we want people to understand in chiropractic. The first twenty-five visits people read these before we check their spine. We ask them what they learned from what they read and let them know their life and health are their responsibility.

Three to Four Yearly Events

We host three to four yearly events designed to take people's understanding of our principles to a higher level. These events are high class. We have live music and amazing food and always make the event a fundraiser. For example, the entrance fee may be a big bag of diapers, which is in turn donated to a local orphanage.

Daily Gems

Our daily communication needs to be quick and concise and get them to think. For example, "David, what exercise do you think I should do?"

"Mary, you are a woman; I am a man. You are thirty-five. I am fifty. You live in your body, and I live in mine. So you and you only can answer this question, Mary. What do you like?"

"I love yoga."

"You see, Mary, all of the answers are within you."

People are sick and tired of having their power taken from them and being told what and what not to do. Empower them through questions and getting them to think. They will love you for it, and you create lifetime relationships.

Monthly Newsletters

We send out monthly newsletters by e-mail, and the topic depends on what is happening in the practice that month. For example, if everyone is asking about pregnancy and chiropractic, then that will be the topic for that month's newsletter. The last six newsletters are printed in the practice all in different colors. We hand the latest ones out always and ask people to share them with others.

> **Without a sense of caring, there can be no sense of community.**
>
> —Anthony J. D'Angelo

PRINCIPLE 7

The Amount of Intelligence in Matter
Autumn Hicks Gore, DC

● ● ●

The amount of intelligence for any given amount of matter is 100 percent and is always proportional to its requirements.

THE INNATE NATURE OF THE world around and inside of us reveals the stories. Natural principles are wonderfully understandable through observation.

This particular principle, describing the perfection of intelligence, has been evident in my life and a light in my consciousness since childhood. I grew up in rural North Carolina, in a quiet, sleepy town, innocently sheltered years behind the modern times. We walked to school, we played outside until dark, and we idolized the legends of our elders. I often spent time in my grandparents' home. I was grateful for their old ears, on particularly adventurous nights when my brother and I ventured out of our beds to creep around the house and explore the completely different world that lived in the dark. When I was about eight years old, my grandpa began to go blind. He was a lifelong welder in a time before there was protection for precious retinas with helmets and goggles. After decades of exposure to literal blinding light, his eyes developed macular degeneration in response to the repetitive stress. Over the next few years, his vision grew darker and dimmer, eventually leading to legal blindness. He was a sharpshooting archer, fisherman, and farmer, and his entire life had been spent on the land he could no longer see. I just remember my heart aching and feeling deep sadness and confusion while thinking, "How powerful could the creator actually be, if he let the world go dark on the wildest man I have ever known."

And then one summer night, in 1989, something unexpected happened. One night, as I crept past his slightly cracked door, toward the kitchen on a path I had taken a hundred times, I heard him call out my name. He *heard* me. He had slept through the same small noises countless nights, but this time, he had not only woken but identified me by the sound of my steps in the black of night. Looking back now, I recognize it wasn't just his hearing that dramatically improved but his sense of smell and touch and even his intuition. As his vision faded, the *intelligence* within his body rerouted, finding other beautifully wondrous ways to express itself. Under his direction, I once drove him to the river, fishing boat in tow, at the ripe old age of thirteen, as he intuitively directed my every turn. Once we got there, he guided me to take the boat to exactly where the fish would be, and I watched in awe as he blindly threaded the fishing lure with precision. The intelligence in his body adapted to the physical changes and limitations and met his requirement…*survival*.

My grandpa's extraordinary rewiring at over sixty years of age wasn't unique to him. I had the gift of witnessing the magic recently in the life of my dear friend, David, a vibrant man full of power and love. After an unexpected illness, simply moving his physical body became challenging, confining him to home and bed, a dim and dark place, just as my grandpa had experienced as his vision slipped away. Then, in the same wondrous way, there was a rerouting. The intelligence of the being in his body found another way out. The expression that he has found in words and language in the last few years has been nothing short of extraordinary. With a limitation in the amount of physical action he can take, he is expressing the same vibrancy and power but now in a completely different way.

It's as if we are submerged in a sea of intelligence. Imagine all matter as unique, beautiful containers submerged and surrounded by this energetic sea. Intelligence fills the body like a liquid that perfectly fills its container. Just like the container, the majority of the human body is empty space, hollow, but permeated by the microscopic light of intelligence that literally fills the space between the actual matter. Like light, intelligence will always find a way—through the cracks, breaks, roadblocks, and U-turns. Intelligence is the core of you, the observer of your thoughts, the adapter of your expression, and the essence of *you*.

You are a human + being. There is a *being* in your human, an intangible intelligence, an invisible energetic glue that permeates matter and organizes its very existence. When something happens *to* you, intelligence in the adaptive force creates the changes that happen with*in* you. Intelligence is always expressed 100 percent within matter.

Our Craft
Damaris-Leigh Lanjopolous, DC, ACP

● ● ●

Top athletes are consummate pros who work obsessively
at their craft. Approach yours the same way.

—Tom Peters

Excellence is not a skill; it's an attitude.

—Ralph Martson

The specific chiropractic adjustment to correct the vertebral subluxation for the full expression of innate intelligence is the heart of our profession. Without this service, we are no different than any other health-care provider. This is what we offer as a doctor of chiropractic.

Is intention enough to deliver a specific chiropractic adjustment? While intention is a large part of how you deliver the adjustment, the skill and specificity in action is in my opinion actually more important. Specificity is the key.

It is far too easy to graduate these days as a chiropractor and be barely able to locate, analyze, detect, and correct vertebral subluxations. Would you want an engineer who graduated from school not understanding the basic philosophy, science, and art of bridge building, building your bridge? Or the surgeon who has spent very little time on actual surgery cutting you open? Wouldn't you want them to be as detailed and specific as possible and have as much training in the actual work that they signed up for?

People are trusting us with their well-being, to do the very best for them. Having criteria by which to assess where the subluxation is, is just as important as correcting the subluxation; otherwise, how can we be sure that we have actually set change in motion?

Consistency and repetition create precision and accuracy. Stick to the same system with each patient to create consistency. We should be focusing on refining our skills, becoming the best adjusters we can be, and delivering those life-changing adjustments that are helping to reconnect man the spiritual with man the physical.

How many times have we heard people tell us that their chiropractor does massage and uses needles and "Oh yeah, he *cracks* my spine too?" The most crucial part of what we do as a profession is referred to as an afterthought, in an almost derogatory way. The patient has not been educated about the most precious gift he or she has been given in the form of an adjustment.

Have you ever had the exquisite blessing of watching a master of a technique in our profession adjust? How amazing is it to see the focus and the specificity and intention and all that goes into delivering that chiropractic specific adjustment. If we are doing anything less, we are surely not living up to the sacred trust that was passed on to us when we accepted our degree as a Doctor of Chiropractic.

> **As the Eagle was killed by the arrow winged with his own feather, so the hand of the world is wounded by its own skill.**
>
> —Helen Keller

PRINCIPLE 8

The Function of Intelligence
Christopher Kent, DC

• • •

The function of intelligence is to create force.

How do you explain this principle to the public?
INTELLIGENCE NEEDS A MEANS TO express itself. Ideas become reality only when set into motion. To express itself, intelligence creates force. In human beings, the nervous system transmits forces between the brain and the various parts of the body. Your heart beats faster when you run or get excited. You perspire when you are in a hot environment.

My first chiropractor explained that chiropractic was based on four simple concepts:

1. The body is a self-healing mechanism. Cut your finger; it heals. Cut the finger of a corpse; it does not. Life heals.
2. The nervous system is the master system of the body. Every aspect of the human experience is processed through the nervous system.
3. When there is interference with the function of the nervous system, not only can it compromise your physical well-being, but it can also have psycho emotional consequences because it distorts your perception of the world and limits your ability to respond to the environment. When this happens to a significant number of people in a society, you have a sick society.
4. What I do as a chiropractor is locate and correct the cause of that interference.

In chiropractic, physical forces are known as universal forces. In living things, they are referred to as innate (inborn) forces.

How does this principle relate to the practice of chiropractic and the correction of vertebral subluxation?

Article 32 in Stephenson's *Chiropractic Text Book* states, "A mental force is that something, transmitted by nerves, which unites intelligence with matter. Mental force is called mental impulse because it impels tissue cells to intelligent action. Mental force is evidently a form of energy, or conveyed by a form of energy, for it can control forces that move matter physically, or balance forces that do it.

The mental impulse, as described by the Palmers, is not synonymous with innate intelligence or the neurochemical action potential. It is a "thought," which may be expressed through a variety of neurobiological mechanisms. The term *mental impulse* was used by D. D. Palmer in his 1910 text. Palmer wrote, "Chiropractors do not treat diseases, they adjust the wrong which creates disease; they have discovered the simple fact that the human body is a sensitive piece of machinery, run throughout all its parts by mental impulse…A mental impulse is an incitement of the mind by Innate or spirit, in the form of an abrupt and vivid suggestion, prompting some unpremeditated action or leading to unforeseen knowledge or insight."

Describing the nature of the mental impulse has been a formidable challenge to students of chiropractic. Early authors were limited by the basic science knowledge and technology of the time. For example, Stephenson wrote, "We might conceive of this mental impulse as being composed of certain kinds of physical energies, in proper proportions, which will balance other such forces in the tissue Cell; as electricity, valency, magnetism, cohesion, etc., etc. Perhaps some of these energies are not known to us in physics. What right have we to assume that we have found them all? The writer presents this as a hypothesis or theory in order to get a working basis…It is no discredit to chiropractic that it must also use theories concerning the transmission of mental forces."

So how does the principle of force and mental impulse relate to the detection and correction of vertebral subluxation? B. J. Palmer employed an instrument known as the electroencephaloneuromentimpograph in an effort to assess mental impulses. Palmer was evaluating the relationship between brain waves, peripheral nerve function, and vertebral subluxation. While we may not be able to measure mental impulses, we can measure and analyze their manifestations. These assessment tools can be used pre and post adjustment and throughout a course of chiropractic care to characterize the neurological changes associated with vertebral subluxations.

- Surface electromyography (sEMG) evaluates patterns of electrical activity in the muscles surrounding the spine.
- Thermal scans assess autonomic function by measuring skin-temperature differentials.
- Heart rate variability (HRV) measures the variations in the heart rate of a patient. chiropractors use HRV to get a window into how the autonomic nervous system modulates heart rate in the baseline or resting state.

Examples of Principle 8 in Action

When intelligence expresses itself through force acting on matter, without interference, the result is normal tone. D. D. Palmer wrote, "Tone is expressed in functions by the normal elasticity, activity, strength and excitability of the various organs, as observed in a state of health. Consequently, the cause of disease is any variation of tone—nerves too tense or too slack...Tone, in biology, is the normal tension or firmness of nerves, muscles or organs, the renitent, elastic force acting against an impulse. Any deviation from normal tone, that of being too tense or too slack, causes a condition of renitence, too much elastic force, too great resistance, a condition expressed in function as disease."

A modern interpretation of tone is tensegrity. Ingber wrote that tensegrity is maintained in "a system that stabilizes itself mechanically because of the way tensional and compressive forces are distributed and balanced within the structure...Cells sense mechanical forces and convert them into changes in intracellular biochemistry and gene expression—a process called 'mechanotransduction.' This work has revealed that molecules, cells, tissues, organs, and our entire bodies use 'tensegrity' architecture to mechanically stabilize their shape, and to seamlessly integrate structure and function at all size scales."

John H. Craven, professor of philosophy at the Palmer School of Chiropractic, wrote, "We have seen that the normal air pressure at sea level is fifteen pounds to the square inch. In order that the body will not be crushed by this weight, it is necessary to have an internal resistance to equal this weight. This internal resistance is maintained in the body by the tone of all of its parts; it is maintained by the expression of mental impulses in the tissue cells."

How does this principle relate to life?

According to D. D. Palmer, "Life is the expression of tone. In that sentence is the basic principle of chiropractic."

Stephenson, in principle 2, stated, "The expression of this intelligence through matter is the chiropractic meaning of life." Principle 8 states the function of intelligence is to create force.

The concept of intelligence creating force to express itself through matter gives a philosophical and physiological basis to an important life lesson. Intelligence must have a means to express itself. Ideas become reality only when set into motion.

REFERENCES

Craven, J. H. *A Textbook on Hygiene and Pediatrics from a Chiropractic Standpoint*. Chicago: Hammond Press, WB Conkey Company.

Ingber, D. E. "The Architecture of Life." *Scientific American* 278 no. 1 (January 1998): 48–57.

Ingber, D. E. "Tensegrity and Mechanotransduction." *J Bodyw Mov Ther* 12 no. 3 (July 2008): 198–200.

Masarsky, C. S., and M. Todres-Masarsky. *Somatovisceral Aspects of Chiropractic: An Evidence-Based Approach.* Philadelphia: Churchill-Livingstone, 2001.

Palmer, D. D. *Textbook of the Science, Art, and Philosophy of Chiropractic for Students and Practitioners.* Portland, OR: Portland Printing House Company, 1910.

Stephenson, R. W. *Chiropractic Text Book.* Davenport, IA: Palmer School of Chiropractic, 1927 and 1948.

Success Formula
Sebastian Carera, Chiropractor

• • •

Defeat is not the worst of failures. Not to have tried is the worst failure.

—George Edward Woodberry

I attribute my success to this—I never gave or took any excuse.

—Florence Nightingale

Sometimes, from an empirical point of view, determining the point of departure can be a great communicational challenge. The question, therefore, arises: *How do I begin?* In my opinion, the best way is to share a *know-how* formula that I have experienced daily—my formula to success.

$$K + S + A^x = \text{SUCCESS}$$

Let us analyze each one of the factors needed to achieve the intended goal. Although the order of factors does not alter the final product, in this case, the order has proven to be a rational and functional way to efficiently achieve the desired result. The first factor, K, represents *knowledge*, the wisdom as such. As human beings, we need a scientific understanding of the phenomenon or cause-effect to be able to get explanations or answers from the theory and practice of our profession. It is the basis for understanding *everything*. Knowledge removes ignorance.. *Knowledge is a necessary element to achieve success.*

The *S* factor represents *skill*—talent in itself. For some people, skill is a "gift" received at the moment of birth. For others, skill means a daily sacrifice to accomplish goals. *The main skill in life is good decision making.* Skill is not inborn. It is learned through repetition and practice.

The last but not the least factor, *A*, represents *attitude*. Our attitude shows the way we cope with everyday life or face certain situations. Attitude is worked out consciously through personal decisions. In this sense, we have two options: we may adopt a gloomy and self-defeating attitude, leading us to negative thoughts and suffering, or we may adopt a positive, cheerful, and dynamic attitude, leading us to hope, to living in the present, and to being happy. *Attitude represents 80 percent of achieving a happy life.*

We, as chiropractors, need *knowledge* to be good professionals. We need to get trained year after year to be updated, improve our techniques, or simply learn something new; we need to know where to make adjustments and where to *not* make adjustments. We need to know the human body, to know how the nervous system works. Without such knowledge and training, we are not good professionals. In my opinion, the only way to grow as a person and as a professional is being ready to learn, being humble, and understanding that every day brings something new to be learned.

Some people think that *skill* is enough to succeed, but if we do not keep our talent, we lose it. Practice and repetition lead to skill. We may have a natural ability for making an adjustment or giving a lecture, but if we do not take some training, it will always still be a "certain" facility. Skill is very important; it makes the difference between a great job and a poor job. *Our achievements depend on us.*

Now, we have to unveil what *attitude* means to us. Unlike the other elements of the formula, attitude is a *multiplying* factor. Without attitude, both knowledge and skill are lifeless. Attitude contains that little spice that makes everything feel wonderful. The main fact is that it only depends on us.

What is success? Success is the point of arrival of many business people, students, and professionals reaching for their dreams. This is our point of arrival too. But when are we being successful? When we have the opportunity to study and train in what we like, when we are able to exercise a choice without coercion, when we may learn with passion, and when we have the opportunity of training for the technique we like best and practicing and continuing to practice to be the best. Nothing appears suddenly. As chiropractic principle 6 says, "All processes take time." We have to work daily to be the best. That is why I am vigilant of the attitude factor, since it is the great enhancer for its capacity to make the difference. Being happy and plentiful or sad and lacking depends on us. Obtaining our objectives and our dreams depends only on us. If we do not practice, we cannot be the best, and if we lack the right attitude we cannot see hundreds of people weekly. Our actions have to be consistent with our attitude. *Our attitude multiplies our results. Study, practice, and be happy.*

Chiropractic has chosen you; take care of it, and respect it.

Before anything else, preparation is the key to success.

—Alexander Graham Bell

PRINCIPLE 9

The Amount of Force Created by Intelligence
Judy Nutz Campanele, DC

• • •

The amount of force created by intelligence is always 100 percent.

PRINCIPLE 9 IS A VERY interesting one. Sandwiched between principle 8 (where force came from) and principle 10 (what force is used for), principle 9 boldly asserts that the amount of force is always 100 percent. Granted, that might not sound like any great thing in 2017 (the time of the publication of this book), when we exaggerate and sensationalize nearly everything. We live in a world where everyone, from an athlete to a salesperson to a spouse, is expected to give 110 percent. We know students with GPAs of greater than 4.0. And we often hear the enthusiastic judges on *American Idol*[1] give a 150 percent "Yes!" Those statements may make sense in a world where everyone on Facebook just had the most amazing weekend *ever*! However, when we seriously and rationally consider the meaning and consequences of the 100 percent in principle 9, it is nothing short of *amazing*!

It would seem to be easier to discuss principle 9 if we first understood what force is and what it does (principle 10). In fact, in his revision of the thirty-three principles, Dr. David Koch suggests that these two principles be rearranged to better facilitate the logical progression of thought.[2] For our purposes, however, we will focus our attention on the *amount* being

---
[1] *American Idol* is an American singing-competition television series.
[2] David B. Koch, *Contemporary Chiropractic Philosophy, An Introduction: A Reformulation of the Thirty-Three Principles and the Normal Complete Cycle* (Roswell, Georgia: Roswell Publishing Company, 2008), 29–30.

expressed. Understand though that force is an immaterial component and for that reason can neither be seen nor measured.

In this context, what does 100 percent mean? First, we have to understand some basic math for this one. (Don't panic you math-a-phobes. I am the daughter of an accountant, but I get the old saying that there are three types of people in the world: those who can count and those who can't!) There are times when percentages greater than 100 percent make sense and are appropriate. For example, you might have 150 percent return on an investment, which simply means that you made back your investment plus 50 percent more! However, when you speak of the entirety of a thing, then of course you could *not* have more than 100 percent.

You could not eat 110 percent of a pie. It is the latter case that applies to principle 9. Stephenson says in his discussion of this principle that "there is nothing to prevent intelligence from creating all it wants…But intelligence being perfect, therefore incapable of incorrect action, creates the requisite amount…the proper amount to perform a specific act—no more, no less—hence one hundred percent."[3] This would suggest that the amount created is not so much a specific quantity as it is the perfect amount or the complete amount. That makes sense too because if force is immaterial and hence nonmeasurable, you could never know if you had it all (i.e., 100 percent of it). Consider a practical application of this principle.

How is it that a rock is a rock and not a stick? A rock is a specific expression of organization maintained in existence by some intelligence. Organization always bespeaks intelligence. We know that because natural laws of the universe indicate that things tend toward disorganization. In physics, we call this entropy, and it is manifested in the second law of thermodynamics. It is the law of universal decay. Yet, a rock is a rock. You can pick it up and roll it around in your hands. There is some intelligence maintaining it in existence as a rock. It does that by creating forces that are expressed through matter that is the rock. If those forces were not 100 percent, it would fail to be a rock.

---

3 R. W. Stephenson, *Chiropractic Text Book* (Davenport, Iowa: The Palmer School of Chiropractic, 1948), 250.

Another significant point to be made regarding principle 9 is that not only does intelligence create perfect force (100 percent), it *always* creates perfect force. That means that not only can it do it, but it does it every time. Consider the pitcher who has a perfect game. That is amazing, and while it rarely happens, it is possible. Now, imagine that extraordinary pitcher having a perfect game *every* time he or she is on the mound. Now, that would be amazing, and that's exactly what intelligence does; it *always* creates the perfect force.

Interestingly, principles 9 and 10 (the amount and function of force) also serve as a pair of principles that correlate with principles 7 and 8 (the amount and function of intelligence). These four principles serve as the foundation upon which the groundwork for the principles of life will be built. Intelligence, force, and matter are the key components to all organization. How these same principles play out in living systems (principles 23, 25, 26, 28, and 31) is particularly exciting and is a significant indicator of the enormity of impact that chiropractic can have on humankind; so keep reading! In the next principle, we will discuss the *purpose* of force, but for now, it is important to know that the *amount* of force created by intelligence is always 100 percent. That is principle 9.

Simplicity
Mary Helen Hensley, DC

● ● ●

Patience, persistence, and perspiration make an unbeatable combination for success.

—Napoleon Hill

Champions keep playing until they get it right.

—Billie Jean King

In 2012 I had a major injury at the same time that my father, who lived in the United States, was preparing to leave this vibration, using Alzheimer's as his ticket home. I had been making the trip from Ireland back and forth to the USA so often that I was on a first-name basis with the USAir pilots and crew on the Dublin to Philadelphia route. I grieved my imminent loss long before my father passed, and it was this injury that allowed me the space and the time to sit with my anguish. It was during this period I discovered beyond the shadow of a doubt that there is a rhyme and reason to all things.

A six-foot-four-inch hulk of a man who played rugby for our local semi-pro team had come to get his spine realigned, following a hard knock on the rugby pitch. After checking him out, I was holding a plastic model of a spine and talking him through the subluxations I had located and was preparing to adjust. I was mid-sentence when I saw this man's giant frame swerve once and his eyes roll back in his head, right before he fell toward me like a giant sequoia felled by a lumberjack. I can't say that anything especially hurt as I hit the floor with 250 pounds of flesh on top of me. The strangest thing was a mysterious noise that distinctly sounded like a piece of paper tearing in two. I yelled out to my office manager, Maureen, as I was pinned under the rugby player and wedged between the adjusting table and the wall, unable to move. Maureen came flying into the room and struggled with all of her might to pull the dead weight off me. As I tried to shimmy my way out from under him, it was then that I realized that something was terribly wrong. The sound of paper tearing had not been my trousers ripping at the seams as I had hoped, but the muscles of my left shoulder literally ripping out of the socket. If only he had remembered to tell me that he always fainted in the dentist's chair at the sight of needles and now upon gazing at plastic vertebrae and rubber nerves.

I will never forget the voice of the doctor who sat down with me following an emergency scan in the hospital later that day. "You're finished," he said, holding the images up to the light. "Yeah, I know," I replied, distraught at the thought of having to get a locum in for a few weeks until I was back on my feet again.

"No, Doc, I think you misunderstood me. You are finished…for good. That shoulder is ripped to shreds. I can't even operate on that in a way that you would ever allow you to adjust again. You're going to have to let it heal on its own, build up scar tissue, and *hope* it will be sufficient enough to provide a bit of stability down the line for limited activity."

To say I was devastated would be to liken a hurricane to a mild breeze. I loved my office and the family of patients I had cared for and nurtured over the last thirteen years. Going to Athlone Chiropractic Care each day had *never* been work.

The long and short of that story is that I have the tenacity of a bulldog and refused to let his grim prognosis become my reality. I used my time to write…seven books so far. I have established myself on the international lecture circuit with some of the biggest names in metaphysics. I have traveled extensively, had a blast with my daughters, pinched pennies, and rebuilt and gotten on with life. Not a moment of time has been wasted. What does this have to do with establishing a successful practice? Allow me to share…

When my resident doc injured himself doing a charity run a few days ago, I had to go in and cover my own practice. I had done it a few times before in the past, a day here or there, knowing full well that my shoulder couldn't handle a full week of work at my old pace of 180 patients a week. A few days, however, I could handle. What made this time so special for me was that I had been asked to write a few words about how to build a successful practice. I was looking at the fruit of my labor of love with different eyes, asking myself all day long, "How did I do it? How did I relocate to a country where I didn't know a soul, buy a practice consisting of thirty active patients, and turn it into a thriving center of love, learning, and living?"

I looked around at the welcoming atmosphere, the approachable front desk, the soothing color scheme, and the shelves full of books on health for young and old. I saw my trusty whiteboard, the same whiteboard that had probably seen ten thousand motivational quotes on health, well-being, and sharing chiropractic with family and friends. I saw the workhorse of an adjusting table, the one that has been recovered a dozen times because the mechanics are so good; the upholstery wears out but the machine never does. I enjoyed flicking through the file cabinets, pulling out index cards—yes, index cards—handwritten, telling more about family holiday destinations, new baby names, achievements in school or sports than about aches and pains. The important and necessary information is all there, but the cards are a testament to years of relying on proficient spinal checks each visit rather than last month's misalignments when considering a person's care. The visits have always been in the now.

I guess what struck me most of all was in the precious few hours that I worked that day, out of nineteen people, only one was a new face, and that's because it was his first visit to the office. So on a random day, I returned to practice in 2017, and every person but the new guy had been with us long before I retired from active practice five years ago. Not bad…

My office manager knows the story of TIC inside and out. She can talk chiropractic better than most chiropractors. She kept the flag flying long after I handed the practice over to my new doc. She gets her spine checked every week, and so does everyone she loves. It's not her job; it's her way of life.

My office isn't fancy; it's clean, welcoming, and educational. The only reason there is a computer in the back room is so my children can do schoolwork and watch videos. Overheads are basic and minimum. It's amazing how much a single office manager can do when there are no insurance papers to file. That's right…we provide a service, and people pay us cash for it. We don't even have a card machine. There's one across the road in the petrol station if someone is really stuck, but no one has ever complained. In 1999, I created the environment in which I wanted to practice. I never allowed the environment to dictate the kind of practice I would have. I educated along the way, through stories, personal examples, and parables of sorts. I never did it all at once, never held anyone hostage until they agreed with my opinion of health, and never took it personally if someone chose to discontinue care. I've never stopped talking about what I do. I never became complacent or lazy. I have remained extremely active in my community. My replacement doc has followed the same path and has immersed himself in the culture, using every opportunity to educate. We have never advertised other than making our presence known on social media (as of late) and an office website. Every person has come to us through referral.

I suppose covering for the last few days has been more of a validation for me than anything else. I was asked about my kids, my mom's health, and my latest book. I talked about little Ronan's Gaelic football match, Catherine's new baby, and Kirsty's graduation Mass. These folks have grown up in my practice and were so well educated over the years that chiropractic simply became a way of life, like exercising or eating healthy. What can I say other than the day was pretty freaking awesome. I can look back at the last twenty years of synergy between my town and my practice and say beyond a shadow of a doubt that we are living the chiropractic dream together.

Energy and persistence conquer all things.

—BENJAMIN FRANKLIN

PRINCIPLE 10

The Function of Force
Shane Walker, DC

● ● ●

The function of force is to unite intelligence and matter.

IT IS MY FEELING THAT the chiropractic principles should not be discussed within a new patient interaction. For example, if I walked into an auto parts store and the attendant began to explain to me the philosophy of changing out a battery and why he sought a career in auto maintenance, I would run for the hills. Just change my battery! However, most practices offer some version of an advanced workshop. Whether it is a spinal care class, progress evaluation, or table talk, these are optimal places to go deeper.

It is difficult to have any meaningful discussion of principle 10 without first considering principle 3, the union of intelligence and matter. This principle states that life is necessarily the union of intelligence and matter. When the triune of life is complete because of force uniting intelligence and matter, an organism has the ability to express its innate potential more fully. This is why the full physiological expression of force is so vital to living systems.

Innate (inborn) intelligence adapts universal forces to be used constructively in the body. With patients, I typically introduce the concept of innate intelligence with a joke. Baby geese don't have to go to school to learn to fly south for the winter; they know how *innately*. Just the same, the body's inborn intelligence knows how to heal a cut and mend a broken bone. However, the body needs a "go-between" to connect that amazing intelligence with the tissues—enter *force*!

In regard to principle 10, the public can easily understand force, as force and energy are terms that can be used interchangeably. When speaking of energy, Stephenson stated, "We might conceive of this mental impulse as being composed of certain kinds of physical **energies**."[4] So now we have a simple understanding that the mental impulse is a force that unites the body's intelligence with its tissues.

Force = Energy = Mental Impulse

Stephenson wrote of two types of forces. *Universal forces* are acting upon the body from outside and are said to be destructive in nature. Examples of these are prolonged sitting, being hit with a rock, and even stress. Stephenson professed that all universal forces are assumed to be harmful to living systems unless deemed otherwise by innate intelligence. For example, it is possible that someone has a fall that inadvertently corrects a vertebral subluxation. It is completely within the realm of reality that a universal force can correct a vertebral subluxation; after all, an adjustment is a universal force! *Innate forces* occur from inside the body and are constructive, acting for the betterment of the organism. A muscle contraction, pumping of blood, and the mental impulse are all examples of innate forces.

Although we typically think of innate forces, such as mental impulses, as subject to being interfered with by vertebral subluxation, universal forces can be interfered with as well. Think of sunlight (universal force) being blocked by a large tree branch casting shade on a forest floor or carrying an umbrella to shield yourself from rain. These are all examples of universal forces being obstructed.

Interference with the transmission of a mental impulse has more significant consequences. There can never be proper health expression without organization. There can be no organization without intelligence. Therefore, when a mental impulse (force) is interfered with, the triune is incomplete. A subluxated body will always result in a lessening of the

---

4 Stephenson, *Chiropractic Text Book*, 268, 269, and 292.

body's innate ability to express health at full potential. As chiropractors, we are continually looking for improved ways to communicate the concept of interference to a mental impulse. Demonstrating the supremacy of the central nervous system is paramount. One simple way is to ask the patient, "How long can you live without exercise? Without food? Without water? Now, how long can you live without nerve supply? Not one second!"

We hold group reports twice a week as an "orientation" for new patients. In the group talk, I walk around the group and hand out a dime to all the participants and ask them to place it on their arm. I ask them if they can feel it, and they all say, "Yes." I tell them to leave it there for a few minutes, and I keep talking. Firstly, this gets them involved not only auditorily but also kinesthetically. Secondly, they are *really* attentive now that this *weirdo* is asking them to set a dime on their arm! After a few minutes, I ask them if they can still feel the dime. Almost always, they say, "No." I then reference Dr. Suh's study at the University of Colorado demonstrating that only ten millimeters of mercury of pressure on a nerve can decrease the "flow" up to 60 percent. Mercury can create interference to the nerve force without the person feeling it.

When patients are face down on the table, I have a captive audience, and it is the perfect time to infuse them with a chiropractic thought. They spend 99.9 percent of their life in the city, at work or school, and plugged into an iPad or television that is inculcating them in an *outside-in* philosophy. The 0.1 percent of their life they are in the office is our opportunity to soak them in an *inside-out* message. People respond well to humor. When they are facedown, I will ask them, "Do you believe in maintenance?"

They will say, "Yes, of course."

I respond with, "Me too! That's why I brush my teeth once a week whether I need it or not!"

Naturally, there is some laughter, but after the adjustment, I bring the point home. "Lifetime chiropractic care is all about communication. If communication within a business or marriage breaks down, this will cause a bankruptcy or a divorce. If there is interference with the nerve force in the body and communication breaks down between parts, this leads to something much more severe—disease. So the reason we hope to adjust you for a lifetime is to allow for full communication in your body so you can be the best you." We just accomplished a few things. We came out first by asking a question. Questions open conversations; statements close them. Next, we used humor to gain attention. Lastly, we used an analogy to demonstrate interference with innate forces.

On a more abstract note, it would be impossible to perceive the concept of intelligence without matter. Intelligence exists in the immaterial and has to have something to manifest within, namely matter. On the flip side, it would be impossible for matter to continue to exist in its essential form without the influence of intelligence. Whether we are talking about a rock or a living system, organization occurs through the application of force by intelligence. Force unites the immaterial and the material, makes the unperceivable perceivable, and unites intelligence with matter.

A peak into the Mind of a Chiropractic Professor
Brian Dooley, DC

• • •

The capacity to learn is a Gift, the ability to learn is a skill, the willingness to learn is a choice.

—Brian Herbert

Tell me and I forget. Teach me and I remember. Involve me and I learn.

—Benjamin Franklin

I HAVE THE GOOD FORTUNE of teaching at Sherman College of Chiropractic. What has become very evident is the fact that the students simply do not know what they do not know. This cause leads to the effect of the perception that the students are missing opportunities that will ensure clarity of vision and purpose upon their graduation date. Would it not be totally amazing if students came out of chiropractic with the personal certainty to rid the world of vertebral subluxations?

As it stands in education, especially chiropractic education, students are hit with a dense amount of material that comes at them with the pace and grace of a firehose. They are forced into a situation in which they must pass boards, and classes are heavily weighted in an area they will use little of in their day-to-day practice. The students come from situations where they say they have been taught chiropractic, but I find myself wondering, have they? Do they realize what they don't know and how that will take their existence as a chiropractor to a level neither they nor their home chiropractor have thought about?

This thought caused me to wonder a bit about myself. What don't I know? What is out there that can make me a better educator, a better teacher, a better chiropractor? In education, the perception is once the class is passed, the knowledge is there, and we move on. As chiropractors, we should always be bettering ourselves. We can start with reading some from the green books to see where the actual mind-set of the discoverer and developer of chiropractic was. Let us discuss with our colleagues consistently to get a deeper handle on the philosophy. Have you ever had an experience where you learned something and said, "Wow, I had no idea about that! How amazing!"? We should all be in a constant pursuit of figuring out what it is we do not know. For if we do, amazing changes will happen to the chiropractic profession at a level none of us can comprehend yet.

What can we do to make this happen? First, we must decide that there is more out there we do not know and now is the time to find it. We can get together with other chiropractors in town who are of like mind and have accountability groups. Create an assignment to read for a week and then discuss. Set up a consistent meeting place and get together to share ideas. Instead of giving health talks on conditions, give them on topics from the thirty-three principles. Titles could be "The cause and effect of your health," "The time Is now for good health," "The universe and you," and "Coordinating your health in a busy world," just to name a few. We should attend philosophy-based events and take thirty minutes to an hour every day to read something on chiropractic. chiropractic has a history of riding the coattails of our leaders from B. J. Palmer to Sid Williams to Reggie Gold to Jim Sigafoose and others. They have done their job; now it is time for us to step up and carry the torch.

Once you stop learning, you start dying.

—ALBERT EINSTEIN

PRINCIPLE 11

The Character of Universal Forces
Edwin Cordero, DC

• • •

The forces of universal intelligence are manifested by physical laws, are unswerving and unadapted, and have no solicitude for the structures in which they work.

IN LIFE, UNIVERSAL FORCES ARE defined across a large spectrum. These forces include those binding atoms together to make molecules, gravity, sunlight, wind, rain, and all the things we eat, drink, and breathe. In life, universal forces are anything, internally or externally, in the physical world that the body of the organism we call human must adapt to in order to not only survive but also thrive. These forces, while created by universal intelligence in the nonphysical realm are manifested, or expressed, as physical laws. They are not false, and they are not broken, even though, at times, people wish they were.

Being that they are physical laws, they work the same every time. Principle 11 states that universal forces are unswerving and unadapted. In life, universal intelligence does not decide which forces work on which matter. Universal forces work on all matter and, as such, are not adapted. Some universal forces may override others, but they are not adapted. For an example of principle 11 in action, think of flying in an airplane. It may seem that the universal force of gravity has changed, or adapted, but it is still there working. Drop something in an airplane, and it will still fall. Gravity is still holding the plane toward the earth; it is just that the universal forces of aerodynamics have over- ridden gravity, at least for a time.

33

Another example of principle 11 in action is how the principle also states that universal forces show no solicitude. Quite simply, as they are physical laws and not physical suggestions. These forces do not care what type of structure they act upon. Universal forces do not care if a sweet, innocent baby or the vilest and evilest human being is in their path. The Internet is littered with film footage of universal forces showing no solicitude. Just think about all the tragic footage showing natural disasters. Whether it be an earthquake in Japan, a tsunami in Indonesia, lightning strikes, or tornadoes in Missouri, universal forces act when the conditions are present for them to reveal themselves. While humans will determine whether an expression of universal forces is tragic, universal forces do not know the definition. They are simply concerned with the building up and tearing down of matter in order to get the universe to a state of entropy.

With respect to how this principle applies to the practice of the analysis and correction of vertebral subluxation, principle 11 is right at the forefront. As previously described, universal forces are unadapted and unswerving and show no solicitude. They work when they want to work and through whom and what they want to. With respect to chiropractic, this includes the human being at the forefront. Universal forces are relentless and continual. In order for a biological organism, like a human being, to remain an active organization as itself, that organism has to adapt to these forces. The biological organism cannot change universal forces. It cannot stop universal forces. Just being nice or doing nice things will not divert the universal forces, which are classified in three categories—thoughts, traumas, and toxins. With a flood of universal forces flowing over and through a biological organism at any given moment, adaption to those forces becomes the key behavior in the survival of that organism.

When the biological organism cannot adapt to these changes, in other words use those forces for its own good, then, in vertebrates, a vertebral subluxation can appear. When the vertebral subluxation appears, it creates a situation in which the biological organism cannot adapt at the ideal rate. If an organism cannot adapt at its ideal rate, there is no way that organism can exist in the ideal expression of its personal innate intelligence. This leads to a less-than organism, which, if extrapolated back to the major premise, leads to a less-than, or decreased, existence of the universe. Think about that for minute.

The fact that lack of adaptation to the internal and external forces that come across, over, around, and through the people of the world creates a less-than world should fuel a chiropractor's fire and desire to make the world the best place it can be with respect to existence. If all human beings were walking down their road of existence in an unsubluxated state, how much better would the world be? How much better would the world be on an individual level? A family level? A country level?

I would explain principle 11 to the public in respect that there are all these forces trying to tear us apart. That is inevitable. What is not inevitable is the state of our existence while we are here. Our bodies have the most amazing ability to use the forces they come across as constructive if they are able to do so without interference. The great thing about universal forces is they are indeed continuous and relentless. Whether we want them or not, they are there. And that is a good thing. We, as biological beings, do not have to worry about generating our own fuel. We simply need to respect and embrace the universal forces around us and convert them into the fuel of our existence. If we want to have the best existence possible for ourselves, our families, our loved ones, and our communities, then we owe it to ourselves and those around us to work the best we can with the universal forces that are all around us. This can only be done with a fully functioning, adapting nervous system free of interference caused by vertebral subluxation.

Certainty of Truth
Chris Zaino, DC

• • •

From principle is derived probability, but truth or certainty is derived from facts.

—Tom Stoppard

Honesty is the first chapter in the book of wisdom.

—Thomas Jefferson

As chiropractors, we don't realize that withholding even 1 percent of the whole truth is lying to that person. I know none of us do it maliciously or with a bad heart; in fact, we actually water down the truth or sometimes even tell little white lies, just to avoid confrontation, keep the peace, keep a relationship together, keep patients from quitting, or persuade a patient to sign up under care. The biggest cause of stress is lying or withholding information (the biggest lie is withholding information).

All animals use deception. Lying is built into our humanity, camouflage to our surroundings. Our humanity is one that leads us to not be 100 percent truthful.

The more you tell the truth, the more you detect your own self-deception and create less stress for yourself and others.

Try the following exercise. Ask yourself, "In which areas have I not been telling the whole truth? Holding back a bit, to avoid creating an uncomfortable situation? What tiny white lies have I told in communication?" Then ask yourself, "*Why* do I do that?" and be totally honest with yourself. This will set you *free*!

Certainty gives you the *edge*. To get the edge, we must be 100 percent certain of what we teach and how we lead. No matter whom the patients know—whether their cousin is a surgeon—if their spine is degenerating daily, choking life off, the disease process progresses daily, killing them. That is not a belief; that is a fact. It is up to them to take full responsibility over that in order to slow it down and stop it ASAP. Your job is just to tell the truth.

> The truth is like a lion; you don't have to defend it. Let it loose; it will defend itself.
>
> —Augustine of Hippo

No matter what they think, subluxation causes degeneration and kills, so whether someone believes it or not does not change the true reality of it.

Ask yourself, "When, where, and why did I or have I lost my edge?" Immersing yourself in the philosophy of chiropractic, in the form of writing, audio, videos, and teaching, on a daily basis, will help you get your edge back!

> **If you develop certainty you can accomplish anything. Even things others say are impossible.**
>
> —Tony Robbins

PRINCIPLE 12

Interference with Transmission of Universal Forces
Caroline Lagerlof, DC, ACP

• • •

There can be interference with transmission of universal forces.

(1) How do you explain this principle to lay people?

I WANT TO MAKE SURE my patients understand and value the importance of the communication between the brain and the body. I explain to them that interruption of this communication is what the medical world uses to determine the event of death, since brain death is the definition of dead. It is through these signals the brain communicates with the body, and the body sends information back to the brain. Without this information, the brain does not know what is happening in the body and can therefore not send out instructions on what needs to be done and how to do it. The information from the right big toe needs to go to the brain without being mixed with other incoming information from the body. The brain needs to be sure it is receiving the correct information; otherwise, the message will be altered and incorrect. It can be compared to when changing frequencies on the radio. The sounds we perceive from the radio are waves transmitted through the air. When altering the frequency on the radio, we alter the waves and thereby the sound we perceive, as the message transferred is different. We will not receive less or smaller parts of the message, just as we wouldn't hear the sound from the radio with lower volume with another type of frequency. As we cannot create the same message without the same type of information, a different message has been formed. Our brain also has a need to fill in the gaps of missing information, without us being aware of it. You can compare it to the filling-in mechanism our brain does with our visual field. The information our brain receives from the eyes is incomplete, partly due to the blind spot and parts of the visual field obscured by retinal vessels, and that is completely normal. We are unaware of this missing information since our brain fills it in, and we perceive the visual field as complete.

In the same way, we as fellow humans have a tendency to fill in missing parts in a story about an episode taking place. Instead of leaving the parts of the story out, where we do not have all the facts clear, we fill them in with what we assume happened in order for it to make sense to us. In the end, we have difficulty knowing for sure which parts we on an unconscious level have composed from an incomplete source of information in combination with our belief and wishful thinking.

Our brain can do its job best if it receives the information without interference; therefore, we must strive for having optimal flow of information through the body.

(2) How does this principle apply to practice and the correction of vertebral subluxation?

Whether we are aware of them or not, we all have principles that create our values in life and which we live by. Some are more aware of these significant factors in their lives than others; despite this, these principles are the foundation for our thoughts and actions.

When you are in your practice working with patients, it is easy to be sidetracked with all the other noise and matters in our surroundings that scream for our attention. As a general rule, in life, it is not the fuss or matters that scream for your urgent attention that make the difference. What is in the core, underneath the surface, where the real matters take place, is where the focus should be.

I don't think you can ask yourself the question "Why" too many times. Whenever I feel I am competent or confident about something, I ask myself "Why?" in order to take it to an even higher level. The "why" question makes me go back to the foundation of what I am doing and the reason for it. In the world we live in, I see it as vital to have moments and sessions where we shut everything else out and focus on the purpose for the work we are carrying out, our "why." When we are clear and have our minds set on this, it will help us implement this intention when we analyze, detect, and correct vertebral subluxation.

(3) Can you give some examples of this principle in action?

Isn't it amazing how well organized nature seems to be? When walking outside in nature, it often amazes me how well thought out everything seems to be, from the big fir trees to the complex ant colonies. It strikes you how everything is intermingled and plays an important role. Even if mosquitos do me more harm than good, their role in the ecological system is important, and when I put my mind to it, I understand how they fill a purpose. However, some parts of nature and its elements are more complex than we humans understand. This does not make them less significant or present in any way. Even though my understanding of how gravity works is far from impressive, it is extremely important, and I wouldn't want to change it in any way. I trust gravity, as well as other aspects of nature I do not fully understand. It does its good even without my fellow humans' and my thorough understanding of it.

Water and different types of water systems are examples of universal forces that have been organized by the universal intelligence to carry out its mission. It is not by chance nature has made them run where they do. Humans have, with different forms of diversions, caused major environmental disruptions. The water systems nature has designed have been interfered with by being blocked and redirected in different forms. Altering a natural habitat, even slightly, can cause a cascade of events that harms the entire ecosystem. Even though it can be difficult and in many cases actually impossible to see the final and overall impact a slight change has on nature, it will not make it less significant and devastating. It will have an impact but in what form?

We then have to ask ourselves the question of whether this alteration is worth the impact and consequence it will have on steps further down the line. We have to try seeing beyond the first, more obvious effect and instead get an anticipation of the overall impact.

(4) How does this principle apply to life?

Universal forces are there, always existing, whether we want them or not, as established in previous principle. At the same time, just as we cannot avoid the universal forces around us, we cannot avoid certain aspects in life. Focusing on avoiding these will not be a winning concept. It is impossible and not the way you want to live your life. It is not the situation itself that is the problem; instead, it's our ability or inability to handle the situation that makes the difference. When something interferes with our ability to handle the situation, it creates imbalance.

We all now and then have situations in life that create negative emotions and stress for us, a bad relationship, for example. As long as we avoid facing the problem and stick our heads in the sand, we will have an inner imbalance. We become uncomfortable and feel wrong when we are ignoring our inner instinct, which I prefer to call *intuition*. A breakup can be devastating, but at the same time, it might be the best thing that could ever happen. What makes the difference is how we react and handle the situation. Either we can see it as a destructive and tough situation and go into a Bridget Jones mode, or we can see through the first dramatic emotions and realize that whatever the reason for the breakup, it would have been damaging to hang on to something creating more negative than positive emotions. It is how we decide to react to and act in the situation that determines the result from it.

> **When we meet real tragedy in life, we can react in two ways—either by losing hope and falling into self-destructive habits or by using the challenge to find our inner strength. Thanks to the teachings of Buddha, I have been able to take this second way.**
>
> —DALAI LAMA

Life is all about going through lessons. They are often tough, but at the same time, they are vital. Despite how big a parent's desire to protect his

33

or her child from all kinds of dangers is, it is quite simply impossible. At heart, the parent understands that it is impossible, and in the end, it would only do more harm than good. As a parent, you want to make your child strong and competent to face life and learn how to handle the struggles that will come in life. You can help your child learn to bicycle with training wheels to start off with, but in the end, you need to take them off and let go for him or her to learn how to find the technique. It is the experiences we go through, both struggles and pleasures, that make us who we are. A parent cannot prepare a child for every single situation that will come in life. It is about developing as many all-round abilities as possible to handle these situations and prepare for life. Our character is created by our experiences of life. It is up to us if we let the lessons in life make or break us.

To Give, to Do, to Love, to Serve

• • •

If you're not making someone else's life better,
then you're wasting your time. Your life will
become better by making other lives better.

—Will Smith

The best way to find yourself is to lose
yourself in the service of others.

—Mahatma Gandhi

When I first saw this motto *on the campus of Life University, I knew my life's purpose had found me. As I listened to Sigafoose talk about what it meant to be a chiropractor and serve thousands of people, every cell of my being filled with energy, life, and meaning. Being called to be a chiropractor has been one of the greatest blessings of my life.*

I had the honor to speak with Dr. Sid for about an hour one day while sitting outside at Life University. He said, "One hand is our business hand, and the other is our service hand, and we must learn how to keep them separate, yet they must be washed together." He said, "Boy, take care of anyone and everyone, regardless of their ability to pay. You will be paid in other ways. Give back. Serve as many people as you can, and the abundance will come and come and come in both financial and spiritual rewards." I will forever value that conversation with Dr. Sid Williams.

The first time I ever stepped foot on Sherman's campus, there was an all-school assembly, and Dr. Thom Gelardi happened to be speaking. Afterward, I went to tell him how much I loved his words of wisdom and that I was seriously considering transferring to Sherman. He said, "David, are you free right now?" I said I was. He then proceeded to take me to lunch and drive me around Spartanburg, talking chiropractic for hours. At the time, he was the president of Sherman and had major responsibilities. Yet he served me and gave to me freely of his time and wisdom, knowing it would impact my life forever.

This message of service must have been instilled in our profession during B. J.'s time period. So many of the great chiropractors that have since passed or are in their eighties and nineties possess this value of chiropractic as a heart-centered service-oriented profession. chiropractic was not a job or a "well-paying profession." Chiropractic was their calling, their life's mission. They never tired of sharing, giving, and serving chiropractic. Many said Gonstead would be in his clinic at all hours of the night and then go and do house calls. This was commitment. To these servants of life, it did not matter if they were being paid or not. Their spirit was flowing through them for a calling much greater than themselves.

If we are going to thrive in practice and as a profession, we must get back to this fundamental principle of service. This is a profession designed for people with heart and a call to something beyond themselves. Chiropractic has the word chi *in it, meaning "life energy." Chiropractic also has the word* chiro *in it, meaning "of the hand." This profession is literally a profession of touch designed to release life-force. That can only be done at the highest level with a heart of service to love, to give, and to do for people out of our own abundance. The beautiful thing is that when you come from this space, you will live a life of abundance. You cannot outgive the giver. This is a universal law.*

No one has ever become poor by giving.

—A<small>NNE</small> F<small>RANK</small>

PRINCIPLE 13

The Function of Matter
Pam Jarboe, DC

● ● ●

The function of matter is to express force.

D. D. PALMER SAID, "TONE is the source, or origin of all life, normal or abnormal. Tone is the element, the source of all life that's quality determines the character of life." A violin exists as matter. Plucking the string introduces a force applied to matter, and the vibration of the string is the expression. The more finely tuned the string, the more beautiful the expression of sound. Quantum physicists discovered that physical atoms are made up of vortices of energy that are constantly spinning and vibrating, each one radiating its own unique energy signature. The nervous system is the modulator of coordinated tone within the body, and when subluxated, it cannot express that tone as well. We are really beings of energy and vibration, radiating our own unique energy signature. People with vertebral subluxation often struggle to express coordination of all body parts and functions, to experience increased awareness, and to evolve in their human consciousness. An individual with less vertebral subluxation is more resourceful at reaching up the rungs of the consciousness ladder to vibrate their unique signature with ease.

EXPRESSING FORCE AS COORDINATING ALL BODY PARTS AND FUNCTIONS

Many years ago, I witnessed an adjustment in which the person stood up off the table and proceeded to violently throw up in the trash basket. My

33

mentor calmly leaned over and whispered, "You'll never see a corpse do that." A few years later, I first heard principle 13 and remembered this story. A corpse is matter. You will never see a corpse cry, laugh, barf, and so on. The power of life is expressing force—life-force. This force just is. It is neither good nor bad, right nor wrong. But often, we observe it as one or the other. We attach a meaning to the expression.

Chiropractors and practice members sometimes view "success" for the patients based upon if they are feeling better. If we adjust them and they feel better, then we have "won" or performed well. We believe chiropractic "works," and we feel validated and powerful. If we get stuck in this way of thinking about winning over the symptoms of the body, then we have succumbed to a mechanistic way of thinking and not relating to a whole being. If we get into this way of thinking, we have forgotten that life is longing to be expressed. chiropractic assists the expression of life and does not try to control it. It is a sacred space to allow another being to express in a world where suppression is considered normal, preferred, and more accepted. The function of matter is to express force, thus allowing for the body to experience "life." This expression may come in the form of fever, vomiting, diarrhea, and so on. We can be open to not judging these things as wrong and needing to be fixed, stopped, anesthetized, and so on. We can choose not to fall into thinking that we are bad chiropractors and we are not adjusting correctly. We can decide that they are not wrong or bad. They are *not* non-compliant. We can stop rejecting people because we think they don't get it. We can be open to a deep knowing that people are not working against us. We do not need to have an adversarial relationship because we are judging their symptoms, judging our abilities or lack of abilities, or judging them. We can step into a clarity of focus that assesses parameters for objectively, measuring nerve interference, choosing the art of when and how to reduce or remove that interference, and then stepping back and allowing life to happen.

This lesson can also be applied to our life and our practice. How often do we judge ourselves or our offices? "This shouldn't be happening." As we often tell patients, symptoms are a wake-up call. Symptoms in our body, in our practices, and in our relationships are an opportunity to become more whole.

Expressing Force as Increasing Awareness

When vertebral subluxations are reduced, efferent and afferent flow to and from the brain are influenced. We are affecting movement of forces to the tissue *and* also influencing information now being shared up to the brain. Patients may possibly experience increased awareness. Things they were dull to before may now become "lit up." They may know so much more about what works and does not work. This is a *very* important process. If a being sits too long and is subluxated, the signals from the body may not reach the brain, sharing that this position is not helpful. After adjustments, the brain may now "get" that this is not in the being's best interest.

One expression of force can be perception. The brain's ability to "read" the internal environment differently is a form of expression. Dr. Candace Pert, author of *Molecules of Emotion*, states, "The way our brain is wired, we only see what we believe is possible. We match patterns that already exist within ourselves through conditioning." An easy conclusion to draw is that as we adjust our patients, their brains change. And as their brains change, they express their life-force in possibly more dynamic ways.

Expressing Force as Evolution of Consciousness

Before most things happen in the physical world, they are conceived in the imagination. My son, Jackson, got confused on the word *imagination* in his early years and used to call it his "magic nation." I found that phrase so much more appropriate and descriptive. In chiropractic, we often acknowledge improved dynamic function on a cellular level and an increased level of awareness but avoid the spiritual evolution conversation.

When people with subluxations get adjusted, their nervous system can often come out of a vigilant, sympathetic dominant state. As a result, there is now someone who's more conscious, aware, and creative. Creativity comes from a spiritual realm, the collective consciousness. The brain (matter) is a receiver, not a source of the force of life, the intelligence that longs to express itself as higher consciousness.

33

D. D. Palmer wrote in the dedication of *The Chiropractor's Adjuster*, "To all those who long to elevate the human race by freeing it from ignorance, traditional prejudice, superstition, and pernicious delusions of the superiority of drug medication and the necessity of surgical mutilation, and especially those who desire to know the best method of removing the unnatural and unnecessary condition known as diseases—conditions which not only cause great suffering, shorten life, and lessen natural and intellectual progress, but prevent proper acquirement of the metaphysical knowledge so necessary for the next stage of existence, this book is most earnestly dedicated." In this one sentence, he encapsulates the concept that the expression of force through matter allows the "elevation of the human race," the removal of suffering from disease, and the acquisition of the metaphysical knowledge necessary for the next stage of existence. As we become less subluxated, we are more capable of accessing the hidden power of our "magic nation" and expressing a higher vibrational resonant frequency. The forces we express in the world as a result of this clear resonance ripple out in waves to all surrounding life.

Practice Management by Objective

• • •

Management by objective works if you know
the objective: 90% of the time you don't.

—PETER DRUCKER

I learned the value of hard work by working hard.

—MARGARET MEAD

THE MOST SUCCESSFUL CORPORATIONS ON the planet are objective driven in their systems, procedures, and outcomes. When you have an objective for each procedure in your practice, your practice will become more reliable, outcomes more predictable, and transition of employees much more effective. I have an objective for every procedure in my entire practice. Here are a few examples:

The First Phone Call
Objective—*to get people into our talk*

Sigafoose was once asked, "If you only had two minutes to explain chiropractic, what would you say?"

His response was "I would use the two minutes to convince them as to why they needed to come and hear my one-hour talk."

Managing by objective gives the assistant a clear understanding that the first phone call is not the time or place to explain chiropractic. The assistant understands very clearly he or she needs to give out only the necessary information to get people into our one-hour talk. The CA understands that if he or she meets the objective on this call, we make more impact in people's lives. Anything less is doing the public a huge disservice.

The First Talk
Objective—*inspire, educate, and empower people to choose to start receiving chiropractic care*

When I first started out in practice and did not understand the idea of having an objective for each procedure, my first talk used to be all over the place. I would teach people about the innate, the difference between health and sickness, how to look at symptoms differently, vertebral subluxations, and on and on.

One day, my CA said to me, "David, let's have a clear objective for this talk. People are inspired, but there is too much information; they are not understanding the basics of why everyone on the planet can benefit from chiropractic!"

This changed my practice completely. I decided to have four events per year where I would teach people deeper concepts of chiropractic and develop a twenty-five-set educational program. This allowed me to focus my first talk on one thing, inspiring them to choose chiropractic care for life.

We redesigned the talk to give basic information about the nervous system, vertebral subluxations, and how we work in our practice. Instantly, we had a huge jump in referrals, and people were following their care plans more consistently and bringing their children more quickly.

Day 1
Objective—*information gathering*
We gather information about the person and his or her vertebral subluxations. This takes place through five concise questions and then a full neural-spinal examination.
Reevaluation

Objective—*reconnection*
We take extra time about every sixteen to twenty visits to reconnect with people about their care. Give them a deeper understanding of what is happening with their vertebral subluxations, reconnect on their plan of care, and reinstate concepts such as the innate or why their children should be checked.

What's measured improves.

—Peter Drucker

Once you have your systems and procedures focused with objectives, it's easy to set up a system to measure how these objectives and systems are working. An example would be the first phone call. If the objective is to get the person into the practice to hear your talk, you can easily measure how many people call for a first visit and how many actually come in to the talk. The results are easily quantifiable, and from that, you can track improvement or identify weaknesses.

I only track numbers and look at things from this viewpoint for one purpose—for our service to be as effective, efficient, reliable, and predictable as possible in order to serve as many people as possible.

Of course, with any heart-centered service, there are always thousands of intangibles that cannot be seen or measured but only felt. Yet the more objective-oriented your systems, the more you can feel the intangibles as well. For example, the number of people referring per week is a sign of an infinite number of tangible and intangible experiences taking place in your practice.

Management is, above all, a practice where art, science, and craft meet.

—Henry Mintzberg

PRINCIPLE 14

Universal Life
Sophie Anderson, DC, ACP

● ● ●

Force is manifested by motion in matter. All matter has motion; therefore, there is universal life in all matter.

How would you explain this principle to a layperson?
THIS PRINCIPLE TALKS ABOUT UNIVERSAL life, but what is that? Firstly, it is important to understand that there is a difference between life and universal life. Life as we generally understand it means something, usually a human being or an animal is breathing, moving around, interacting with others, and adapting to the world within which we live. We also recognize that plants, trees, and even bacteria are alive and therefore have "a life," or a life span, a period of time during which these things express life.

How do they express life? It is very easy to see in a human being or animal. Not only do we visibly breathe and move around, we also have many complex systems and processes occurring internally every second. These highly complex and organized signs of life are orchestrated by an innate intelligence. It's important to note that "intelligence" in this instance is different from the "consciousness" that we consider intelligent life forms to have.

See principle 20 to learn about innate intelligence. Examples of these signs of life include our ability to extract what we need from our environment through breathing, eating, or drinking and then excrete the waste or toxic by-products that we do not require. Additionally, we have the ability to reproduce and therefore ensure the continued existence of our individual species, as well as constantly adapt to our external environments. All of these qualities are also carried out, just in less obvious forms, by plants and even bacteria, which are invisible to our naked eye.

Although there is clearly life in bacteria through to human beings, it is obvious that they differ in the complexity of their structures and functions and therefore how much organization or order is required. In contrast to life, we can easily recognize when a human being or animal has died despite the physical presence remaining the same in the first moments following death. In a state of death, the dead do not express signs of life; they are no longer running the same systems and processes that were so beautifully orchestrated during their life-span by innate intelligence. *Life* has left their body; however, something is still holding them intact, at least initially. This is one example of universal life. Let's look at what that means. To fully understand universal life, firstly, we need to distinguish what we mean by the word *matter*. In the previous example, the physical parts of a human body are one example of matter. At school, we also learned about gases, liquids, and solids; these are all different forms of matter. We know that solids have a distinguishable shape, and we can usually pick them up or touch them. Liquids are more fluid and adapt to the container that they are in while still being visible, whereas we struggle to see the majority of gases with our naked eye.

We also learned that different materials or types of matter could change form. For example, liquid water can freeze into solid ice just as easily as it can evaporate into a gas that we no longer see. Science experiments allow us to capture this invisible gas and convert it once again into liquid water. Therefore, just because we cannot see the gas does not mean it does not exist. It is just in a different form from what it was when it was a liquid or a solid.

What is holding these structures together or allowing them to change form (even when we can't see them)? At school, we were told there were bonds between the building blocks or molecules of all things; we pictured these bonds as a physical tie between one molecule and another. We now know that actually these bonds are an invisible force, much like gravity, and these, along with the molecules, are moving constantly; in fact, they are vibrating.

Depending on the rate or speed of vibration of these bonds, the matter will change its form. Solids, liquids, and gases all have differing rates of motion or vibration in their bonds. Without this vibration, the building blocks just would not be held together in the same way, and the object or matter would take an entirely different form or even cease to exist. This vibration, or motion, is essential to organize or maintain order in all the matter in our universe, whether it be a solid, liquid, or gas. There is no such thing as zero movement in our universe, and this motion exists in all things, whether they are living or nonliving.

In living things, as we already discussed, there is an additional layer of organization provided by the presence of an innate intelligence. In non-living things, such as a car tire, water in a glass, or helium gas within a balloon, they are still clearly organized in some way and held together by these invisible, moving bonds.

It is this organization, in all matter, provided by these invisible moving bonds, whether it be living or nonliving, that tells us that within our universe there is order. In the simplest possible way of explaining it, universal life is order or organization.

How does this principle fit into practice and the correction of vertebral subluxation?

As we outlined in the past section, there is organization or order in everything in our universe, living or nonliving. Everything is maintained in its state of existence by the motion or vibration of the bonds and building blocks from which it is made.

Within living things, the state of organization is higher, more complex, than in nonliving things. This complex level of organization and adaption is orchestrated by innate intelligence. In vertebrates, that is, humans and animals with a nervous system and spine, it is recognized that innate intelligence communicates through the nervous system.

There exists the possibility of changes to the normal movements, or biomechanics, of the moving parts of the spine. These abnormalities directly change and hinder the normal function of the nervous system, because of the close proximity of the spine, spinal cord, brain stem, and nerves (the spine is the house of the nervous system) and the way they are *wired*.

Altered biomechanics of the spine result in altered nervous-system function, which can lead to an altered ability of innate intelligence to do its job. In this event, known as vertebral subluxation, there is a negative impact on the complex organization of all the life processes that each human being carries out second by second. Not only is the normal movement of one or more segments of the spine lost, but consequently, normal motion or vibration between the molecules and bonds of the body (the physical parts of the body) is absent. As previously discussed, differing rates of motion and vibration lead to a change in the form of the matter (think of the differences between gases, liquids, and solids). It is widely accepted within science, design, and even architecture that "form determines function." The differing form or expression of matter therefore changes its function. In simple terms, this means that the cells and different building blocks of the body cannot behave and adapt in the way that they were designed to. Their design is not faulty; it is the controlling intelligence, which is no longer in charge.

Think of the cells in the body like children in a classroom and the innate intelligence like the teacher. With the presence of the teacher, structure and order remain. As soon as the teacher leaves the classroom for a period of time, chaos ensues. None of the desired outcomes are achieved, and generally a large majority of the children (cells) start misbehaving; they could even start doing themselves or each other harm.

Less organization and order in the body not only affects what is happening internally but also equates to less ability to process and adapt to the external environment. A reduction in the ability of innate intelligence to do its job alters the balance between its inherently creative quality for the overall good of the individual and the external forces of the outside world, generally deemed as destructive.

Without this balance between organization and creation versus destruction, destruction takes over, and things start to break down. On a day-by-day basis, this could result in a whole array of changed functions. Who knows how far reaching these consequences are. We can only presume based on the facts we know and logical deduction that this could impact all facets of their lives from their ability to run their internal systems of digestion, reproduction, and respiration to how they perceive others around them and the relationships that they have and create.

Over an extended period of time, this reduced ability to coordinate repair and restoration of all physical (solid) parts of the body can ultimately lead to early breakdown of the physical matter of which we are made. It is logical, therefore, that that particular human being will express life for a shorter period of time than he or she was designed to. Correction of vertebral subluxation through specific chiropractic adjustments restores normal movement to the spine and function to the nervous system, allowing innate intelligence to do its job: organize for the greater good of each individual within which it resides. With greater organization comes greater adaption and therefore expression of life. Simply put, vertebral subluxation impedes organization and therefore our expression of both life and universal life.

On the contrary, correction of vertebral subluxation allows restoration of organization (universal life) and the ability of innate intelligence to create order and therefore expression of life. It adds life to our years and years to our life.

How does this principle fit into life?

In the grand scheme of life, we understand that motion is life; if we are not moving, we are dying. Modern-day health campaigns are even stating that that sitting is the new smoking, when talking about the damaging effects that a lack of movement has on our human experience. This principle reminds us that motion is essential to all life and everything that exists within our universe down to the very smallest particles. Without motion, nothing would exist in the way that we know it. Additionally, without normal motion of our bodies and spines, everything changes in function, which can have far-reaching effects on our human experience.

Can you give examples of this principle in action?

This principle is beautifully demonstrated by the changes we see when gases change to liquids and liquids change to solids and vice versa as we discussed in the first section. In addition to this, we can see universal life in a dead leaf that has fallen off a tree. Just because it is dead does not mean it ceases to exist. The principle of universal life explains why it still remains intact, because of the motion in the solid matter of the leaf.

Servant's Heart
Christopher Wolff, DC

● ● ●

> To give real service, you must add something which cannot be bought or measured with money, and that is sincerity and integrity.
>
> —Douglas Adams

> The best way to find yourself is to lose yourself in the service of others.
>
> —Mahatma Gandhi

THE NUMBER-ONE FACTOR GOING INTO chiropractic practice I believe is showing up every day with a servant's heart. It really goes for any service, but I feel especially for this profession, a servant´s heart is essential to have success and longevity. Getting motivated to do anything can be helpful, but it usually doesn't last. The reason for this is that it comes from the outside in, and unless that motivating factor strikes something to inspire us from within, it will eventually die out. All of the highly successful chiropractors I know deeply love what they do and deeply believe in it. It isn't just a job that they sought out to make good money. In fact, I could argue that abundance of money wouldn't be there unless they had the passion and inspiration to hustle every day. To serve and assist their communities express life and health more purely through the location, analysis, and correction of vertebral subluxations.

I also find that many chiropractors, and more so today, treat this career as a hobby—like it's what they're going to do Monday, Wednesday, and Thursday. I believe one of the prevailing reasons for DC's failing is not taking this seriously as a business and running it as such. Having systems in place for management is crucial to success and reproducibility as is knowing all of the business numbers. A program into which you can enter business statistics to keep track of your daily, weekly, monthly, and yearly progress is crucial; it's like the saying, "What gets measured gets managed." As chiropractors, our calling is to serve people, and if we don't manage our business properly and closely, we can't do this as effectively or efficiently—or, in the worst case, at all.

Many chiropractors I have talked to over the years have had a fear of marketing or just no idea what to do, period. I think a lot of times we over think things and instead of just doing something or anything, we end up doing nothing. I believe that thinking is overrated and doing is very underrated. No one is good at everything, but we are all good at something(s). Figuring out your strengths and weaknesses is crucial in determining what kind of marketing you want to do. Whether it is social-media campaigns, screenings, talks, or health fairs is not important. What is important is that you find the ways that work for you to get your message and brand out to your community, so that they can find about your office and services. This process takes a lot of time and persistence, so patience is essential—microspeed and macropatience.

> **Service to others is the rent you pay**
> **for your room here on earth.**
>
> —MUHAMMAD ALI

PRINCIPLE 15

No Motion without the Effort of Force
Daniel Facchini, Chiropractor

● ● ●

Matter can have no motion without the application of force by intelligence.

How do you explain this principle to the public?
BY KNOWING THAT THE FUNCTION of intelligence is to create force (principle 8) and that the function of force is to unite intelligence and matter (principle 10), we can deduce that all motion is a consequence of force acting through intelligence. This means that all motion occurs as a consequence of the same intelligence that maintains matter in existence and, ultimately, maintains our body in equilibrium.

All the actions throughout the universe are caused by motion. It is heartening to see the designs of intelligence in every existing action, permeating reality inexorably with active organization.

Uniting deductive reasoning to the accumulated knowledge created by the inductive method can be an enriching endeavor, since we can verify observable phenomena and use them as yardsticks of the deductive path traveled by reason. Thus, we create premises, and we put them to the test.

Advances in different scientific areas have demonstrated that isolated analysis of variables does not allow a more comprehensive conception of reality. This can be seen in two striking examples: the limit in the acquisition of all the information related to a particle, determined by Heisenberg's uncertainty principle, and the manifestation of emergent properties (as described by Lewes).

In this light, we need to understand the motion of any fragment of matter as a motion embedded in a larger context: relative motion. There are no means, be they rational or empirical, to determine whether we are in motion, except through our *relationship* with another fragment of matter. This relativity encloses motion into a holistic network, in which forces become relevant only as a cause of it, and intelligence assumes its universal character by creating this web of relations, permeating all matter and energy.

The term *energy* is used here as a capacity to do work. From a purely deductive point of view, we could consider it interchangeable with the force because of its capacity to generate motion. However, it is known that energy and matter are aspects of the same entity and can be transformed into one another, energy being equal to the product of the mass of matter times the speed of light squared.

In a nutshell, all motion is the result of the force created by intelligence. Motion matters only in relation to something, and this relationship allows us to understand the unity of the whole universe under the mantle of organization orchestrated by intelligence. Finally, it is interesting to realize that the reverse path is also true: intelligence exists through the expression of force, perceptible through relative motion.

How does this principle contribute to the practice of chiropractic and the correction of vertebral subluxation?

When we understand the subluxation as a disturbance in the active organization capacity of the individual, we can regress, using deductive reasoning, back to the importance of intelligence in the organization of matter and its determining effect on its motion. Through this method, it is plausible to think that the presence of a subluxation may potentially have a negative influence in the motion that intelligence would designate for matter if it could act without interference.

Moving beyond this plain line of reasoning, perhaps it is even more interesting for us to think in the opposite direction: the existence of intelligence as an expression of the force perceivable through motion. In this view, if the nervous system is what expresses an adaptive intelligence for the body, a subluxation could be understood as a limitation on this connection between them, rendering it impossible for innate intelligence to recognize the state of bodily matter. This lack of information hampers the system, since it has to work with insufficient information. It is a two-way relationship.

Can you give some examples of this principle?

The study of motion has been a fertile field of investigation over the millennia. In antiquity, the Greek philosopher Aristotle proposed that the elements moved by seeking their natural place of rest. Thus, objects would fall because they were attracted to their resting place, which was the closest possible to the center of the universe (which, at that time, was thought to be the very center of the planet earth), and they would not move from there until another force acted on them. The hypothesis that the natural state of motion is to be at rest is incongruent with the law of inertia, proposed hundreds of years later by Galileo and Newton. The fifteenth chiropractic principle does not contradict the law of inertia, if we accept that the force is necessary to generate motion but, once generated, it will remain unchanged forever, until another force acts upon it. Thus, a moving object may well have no force influencing it at any given moment, but it carries with it, through its direction and velocity, an information of the force (and therefore of the intelligence) that affected it in the past.

We can derive another example, this one from deductive reasoning alone. It points to the fact that it is impossible for intelligence to exist where matter has no motion. Since the two are inseparably connected by force, the stillness of the universe would imply the total absence of forces acting on matter and, consequently, the complete absence of intelligence.

How does this principle relate to life?

When we consider *life* as the expression of intelligence through matter (principle 2), it is clear that motion is the only expression of universal life that is perceptible to us. We cannot directly deduct intelligence. Even Strauss (in *Chiropractic Philosophy*, 1991) mentions that a leap of faith is necessary for the acceptance of the major premise.

Regardless of the acceptance of the universal intelligence construct, it is grounded in the observation of motion. And curiously, the ability to observe motion could guide us to an *a posteriori* premise from which the

33

first could be deduced: there is motion. If there is motion, there is force. If there is force, there is an agent that causes this force. And as we do not identify this agent, we can adopt the working hypothesis that there is an intelligence that generates the force.

The analysis of the opposite end of this reasoning process helps us to confirm the relationship between motion and life; stasis implies universal death within a deductive standpoint. Where there is no intelligence, there is no life, there is no organization, there is no force, and there is no motion. There is only nothingness, darkness, and emptiness.

Love what you do and do what you love

• • •

Choose a job you love and you will never
have to work a day in your life.

—Confucius

Success is no accident. It is hard work, perseverance,
learning, studying, sacrifice, and most of all love
of what you are doing or learning to do.

—Pele

Love what you do, and do what you love. In my opinion, there is no greater key to success than loving what you do with every fiber, cell, and tissue of your being. People will be attracted to you like magnets. Your passion and energy will become contagious. Think about it. How many people do you meet each day who unequivocally love what they do beyond words?

When you love what you do so much that it becomes one of your greatest hobbies and joys, life becomes an endless vacation. Since I was called to be a chiropractor, I never worked a day in my life. It's as if I have one of the most precious gifts on earth, and the more I share it, the more abundant and rich my life becomes, both materially and otherwise.

33

When you love what you do, you will take action to share it with others. No one will have to force you to get out of bed each day. Life seems to conspire in favor of those people who love what they do. It is truly vitalism in action. There is a deeply spiritual essence moving through the person who loves what he or she does. His or her work flows and is anything but mechanical. The heart and soul shine through the person who loves what he or she does beyond measure.

> **The universal force is love. When scientists looked for a unified theory of the universe they forgot the most powerful unseen force.**
>
> —ALBERT EINSTEIN

PRINCIPLE 16

Intelligence in both Organic and Inorganic Matter
Joe Strauss, DC, FCSC

•••

Universal Intelligence Gives Force to Both Organic and Inorganic Matter

PRINCIPLE NUMBER 16 HAS THREE critical components. Look at it again. Universal *intelligence* gives *force* to both organic and inorganic *matter*. Intelligence. Force. Matter. Sound familiar? It should. It should remind you of principle 4, the triune of life. Life is a triunity, having three necessary united factors, namely: intelligence, force, and matter. Principle 4 is the first time all three components are mentioned together. Then, of the next twelve principles up to and including 16, all but three (principles 6, 11, and 12) discuss the relationship and relevance of these components—intelligence, force, and matter, in one way or another. One of the critical distinctions of principle 16 is the introduction of the term *organic*.

To be clear, it should be noted that *organic* might not be the preferred term today. If we could, we might rewrite this principle to read, "Universal intelligence gives force to both *living* and *nonliving* matter." We have to understand that any historical writing must be viewed in the time in which it was written. That's why Bible scholars must understand Greek, Hebrew, and Aramaic. In 1927, the developers of our profession did not write in Hebrew and Greek (although sometimes it may seem like it), but B. J. Palmer and R. W. Stephenson understood the words *organic* and *inorganic* differently. At that time, the terms differentiated living and nonliving matter. Language changes constantly. My late father-in-law was

33

a professional magician. When he first went into the profession, he called himself "The Gay Deceiver." He eventually had to drop that moniker because the meaning of the word *gay* changed during his lifetime. Today, we define organic and inorganic matter to differentiate that which has a carbon-hydrogen-oxygen bond and that which does not. Consider that a tree alive in the woods and a front door made out of that same tree would both be classified as organic matter; however, one would be living and the other would be nonliving. For this reason, principle 16 might be better understood if written as "Universal intelligence gives force to both *living* and *nonliving* matter." So what's important about the introduction of the concept of living matter in principle 16?

We already know that the function of intelligence is to create force (principle 8) for the purpose of uniting intelligence and matter (principle 10). We also know that the function of matter is to express force (principle 13), that force is expressed in matter as motion (principle 14), and that matter cannot have motion without the application of force by intelligence (principle 15). These principles explain how matter, up to this point *nonliving* in nature, is maintained in its unique expression of existence—why a chair is a chair and a shoe is a shoe and a rock is a rock. After principle 16, the discussion is directed at *living* things, and the concepts and relationships of intelligence, force, and matter as found in living things. Principle 16 is the necessary logical step to connect these two separate and equally important, distinct types of matter. However, principle 16 says universal intelligence gives force to *both* organic *and* inorganic matter. This is the other critical distinction of principle 16. Palmer explains, "If Universal Force is universal, which it is, it is impossible for any mater to be where Universal Force is not." That includes organic matter as well as inorganic matter, or in today's language, living matter as well as nonliving matter. The inquisitive student might ask how that could be when we know that it is innate intelligence that gives force to living matter as described in the latter half of the thirty-three principles.

Let's look more closely. The forces that maintain the electron of a carbon atom in organization are universal forces. However, when that carbon atom makes up the cell structure of a living organism, these universal forces are then adapted by the innate intelligence of the organism. If the cell is removed from the organism, then the innate intelligence of the cell takes over the responsibility of adapting those universal forces for the good of the cell. When it can no longer do that, the cell once again becomes universal matter and is organized on the molecular level via universal intelligence. It is again subject to universal forces.

Universal forces are the expression or manifestation of existence and can neither be created nor be destroyed. All matter expresses existence, whether it is living or nonliving. Living matter expresses innate intelligence as well, and it manifests one or more of the signs of life. A corpse no longer expresses the forces of innate intelligence, but it still has existence as a corpse. Even when it becomes dust, it still has existence. In fact, the same chemicals exist in a living human being, a corpse, and the dust it becomes; they are just being expressed differently. In fact, the same chemicals exist in a living human being, a cow or a carrot, a corpse, and the dust or soil they become. It is just matter being expressed differently.

We can use the laws of gravity and aeronautics as analogies to better understand the principle. Both laws are in existence all the time. While a plane is flying at thirty thousand feet, only the law of aerodynamics is being expressed; however, the law of gravity does not cease to exist. The law of aerodynamics requires power so it would be analogous to the law of life (innate intelligence). The law of gravity, analogous to universal intelligence, is still there; it's just not being expressed or manifested. As soon as the power is shut down or cut back, the law of gravity, while always present, now begins to be expressed. We could carry this analogy further and liken the cutting back of power to a vertebral subluxation and liken the engine totally being shut down to death. The difference is you cannot restore life (innate intelligence) to a totally dead body (except in Frankenstein movies). When the plane is on the ground, only the law of gravity is manifested until the power is restored and the plane takes off again. Meanwhile, the law of aerodynamics is still in existence; it is just not being expressed.

We will learn of the specifics of the expression of intelligence, force, and matter in living things in subsequent principles. For now, principle 16

33

is ideally placed as a bridge between the concepts and relationships of intelligence, force, and matter in nonliving things, discussed in the first fifteen principles and how those concepts and relationships are expressed in living things and their ultimate significance to chiropractic and humanity, as will be discussed in the principles that follow. It is the next logical step in the progression of our chiropractic principles. Universal intelligence gives force to *both* organic and inorganic (i.e., living and nonliving) matter.

Levels of Conciousness
Jane Burnier, Chiropractic Assistant and Life Coach

• • •

The key to growth is the introduction of higher dimensions of consciousness into our awareness.

—Lao Tzu

No problem can be solved at the same level of consciousness that created it.

—Albert Einstein

There are four basic levels of consciousness and places to come from in your office. Each of these places within ourselves creates a different outcome in our experience and the experience of the people we serve.

The first level of consciousness is survival. In this place, we are asking ourselves, "How am I going to pay the rent? Who is the competition down the street, and what are they doing? How many new people do I need to get this month? I wonder how good their insurance is." You may ask people questions in that first visit such as "Where is your pain? On a scale of one to ten, how bad is that pain? Does the pain increase when you raise your arm? How long do you want to suffer with this pain?" You have spinal degeneration pictures on the wall, and you scare people into signing up for an extended period of care based on fear. You tend to talk about the latest news in the world or the weather or politics. The energy in the office is dense and often sterile.

At the level of survival, you live as a victim, so you will attract others who feel victimized as well. You attract people who do not take responsibility for their own health and only want relief from symptoms. Once the symptom is gone, they are gone as well, leaving you to constantly look for new people to fill your day. Your internal dialogue is "People just don't get it."

From that place, we give them survival conversation and education. "You have phase-three spinal degeneration. You have a silent killer in your spine just waiting to suck your life out."

Your conversation is fear based and control based. You have people call you "doctor," and you might even wear a white coat. You have pictures on the wall of spinal degeneration. You feel stressed, and your energy field impacts your "patients." Life is a constant struggle. From this level of consciousness, you are manipulating the spine.

Level 2 is logic. From this place, you just want to figure everything out. You are completely in your head. The message you give is you have a brain that controls the body through your central nervous system; if there is a subluxation in the spine, it cuts off nerve supply to your organs, and those organs will eventually begin to fail, leading to symptoms and eventual death. You show them the spinal charts and how this nerve when subluxated creates a certain symptom. It is a mechanistic model of practice. You will attract other logical people who will plague you with all kinds of questions about research, double-blind studies, and so on. They want proof and statistics. This is a very draining way to practice.

The people you attract live in their minds and are not very likely to refer or to remain under care once their symptoms have decreased. In this type of practice, you have to constantly do spinal screenings and other marketing endeavors in order to keep the practice afloat. There is little joy to practicing this way. At the end of the day, you are drained. You are competent but not masterful. You are a servant at this level, meaning you give from your need to please or your need to be needed.

Level 3 is synchronicity. At this level, your will and the will of god are in alignment. Your interactions are about the people you are serving. You genuinely care about them and their life's journey. You are asking them questions about themselves and really listening at a level that validates their experience without judgment; you have no agenda to "get" them. There is no fear, no convincing; you speak truth from your heart. You may ask them, "How will your life change once you have regained your health?" You attract people who are open and loving. They get the big picture and refer others because they realize that you don't have to be sick to get well. Your office is a place of healing. You have toys for the children and uplifting reading material. You give inspiring talks, and you walk your talk. At the end of the day, you feel connected and satisfied with your service. You serve, but you are not a servant. Service comes from your own abundance, the deep wellspring of life. Being a servant comes from a need to please and is very draining.

Level 4 is the consciousness of love. Your complete trust in universal wisdom is pouring out of every cell of your body. You are congruent with your message, and you bring your entire being to the conversation. You listen deeply with presence, and you are able to access the innate wisdom of your clients just by being open and receptive to their experiences. Your conversation is completely based in truth, trust, acceptance, and presence.

Your conversation is about potential. You educate your clients to understand the greater truth and idea of who they can be in the world when they are free of nerve interference. You are inspiring, open, and an example of a true human being. You are living your potential. Your office is filled with pictures of children who are being checked and cleared. You have beautiful art that expresses the beauty and wisdom of nature and life. Your waiting room is filled with families. You have created a fee system that is congruent with lifetime care. You really love the people you serve. At the end of the day, you feel energized and full of life and optimism. You speak very little while practicing, and everything you say is about innate wisdom and universal wisdom.

Your people refer others and bring their families. You are abundant financially, and your nervous system is at ease. You are a master, as you have created your own technique, adding your own innate abilities to your adjusting skills. You are confident, and you are able to let go of anything that does not serve you. At this level of consciousness, your café becomes a beacon of light. You are aligned with the source, and the life-force becomes your partner. The people you attract operate at a higher level of consciousness, and once they understand the power of innate wisdom, they begin to blossom. They may continue to have symptoms, but they understand that having a clear nervous system is what is really important.

Have you ever noticed that when you go to certain seminars when you return to your office, you have a burst of new people and people coming back in to get adjusted? Why? When we go to seminars such as this, our state of consciousness increases. A person will never seek out a healer with a lower level of consciousness than his or her own. So when your state of consciousness increases, so does your practice. But as weeks go on, many people tend to slip back into their old thinking and the people begin to disappear.

The higher the state of consciousness that you can hold, the more people are available for you to serve. So your real work is to have an open heart, wonderful adjusting skills, an openhearted and educated chiropractic assistant, a fee system that encourages ongoing care, and the consciousness of love.

How do we stay in that state of love? Ask yourself three questions when you feel yourself slipping into lower states: "What do I need to let go of, or forgive, in this moment? What or whom do I need to accept right now? What can I trust in this moment?" Asking yourself these three questions immediately shifts your state of consciousness.

As a chiropractor, you have a choice to make: you can either come from ego, fear, and powerlessness, or you can come from love, potential, compassion, and openness. Healing occurs in the presence of presence.

Our greatest contribution to humankind is to serve them with love and integrity. Our greatest need in practice is how to add value to their life.

The single purpose of a chiropractor is to make sure every man, woman, and child within his or her realm of service lives a subluxation-free life. The innate intelligence from within them will guide their path to abundance and health. Our role there forth is to keep them clear, connected, and accountable.

> **Remember your perception of the world is a reflection of your state of consciousness.**
>
> —Eckhart Tolle

PRINCIPLE 17

Cause and Effect
Lona Cook, DC

● ● ●

Every effect has a cause, and every cause has an effect.

How would you explain this principle to the public?
THE SEVENTEENTH PRINCIPLE IS "CAUSE and effect"—every effect has a cause, and every cause has an effect. This principle is important in our understanding of the bigness of our connection in our universe. We are all interconnected and intertwined through the energy present in this universe that we are part of. We are made of the stuff of the universe. Quantum physics is studying the vibratory nature of our connection through quantum entanglement. In simple terms, every moment, action, thought, and so on affects the whole. A cause or change in one part of the universe ripples and has effects in the rest of the whole; the system must operate collectively, because at a quantum level, it is all vibrational energy. This is also why our own personal evolution and adaptation to wholeness as beings profoundly affects our world.

How does this principle relate to practice and the correction of vertebral subluxation?

This principle is important for our chiropractic work because it furthers our understanding of what it is to be *alive* (and connected into the universe). We are not machines; we are energetic beings with material and nonmaterial aspects. Vertebral subluxation exists because it is an effect of the being's inability to fully process in that moment, creating the effect of subluxation in the nervous system and being's energy. It is an adaptation as a protective feedback.

This effect of vertebral subluxation leads to further effects in those physical, mental, emotional, and spiritual states of the individual and the greater world because of the entanglement of all beings through our energy fields. This is why the correction of vertebral subluxation and the innate's ability to reprocess the subluxated energy causes an effect of a shift back toward wholeness, and that restoration ripples off for many positive effects in that being and in the universe.

How does this principle relate to life?

This principle is life; it's when you wake up to know you are more than the sum of your parts. It's when you know your brother, neighbor, and strangers are parts of the greater you. It's how you begin to choose better for yourself and move toward healing and wholeness for yourself and to see shifts in all aspects of your outer world, because we *are* all connected through this principle of cause and effect.

This principle encompasses big thoughts about the universe that many of us were not taught as we grew. So here is a quick story to illustrate this principle.

A cause can come in many forms. In my story of a man named Gabriel, the cause I choose to focus on starts with a series of chiropractic adjustments given to a man during a mission trip in the Dominican Republic. Gabriel had suffered a stroke nearly two years prior and was confined to a wheelchair. He also had paralysis of his arms and hands. After receiving several adjustments to his atlas vertebra in an afternoon, he was able to stand, lift his arms, and move his hands. It was a profound moment of seeing the reconnection of the innate and a man's physical body through chiropractic care.

However, the story doesn't end there; it continues to ripple off, becoming a cause for more effects. I had the pleasure to share this story in the United Kingdom at a chiropractic seminar. After the seminar, a DC came to me and thanked me for sharing the story of Gabriel. I didn't think twice about it and flew back to the States. Weeks later, I received thank-you letters in the mail from patients in London who had suffered strokes and were now under chiropractic care and having great healings. They were thanking me for sharing the story of Gabriel because it had impacted their chiropractor to start checking their spine more often and was creating change and healing for them on a new level. I had no idea that would happen.

Interestingly enough, I also realized that before I had left for that Dominican mission trip, I had written a goal to "see a chiropractic miracle." And that trip is when I met Gabriel and had a chance to watch his healing. As you can see, there are many causes and many effects, and as B. J. Palmer said, most of the time, we will never know how something we think, say, or do will affect the lives of millions tomorrow. The law of cause and effect is an important one for us all to recognize in our existence.

Explode Your Practice
Steve Judson, DC

• • •

Keep your dreams alive. Understand to achieve
anything requires faith and belief in yourself, vision,
hard work, determination, and dedication. Remember
all things are possible to those that believe.

—Gail Devers

Leadership is the capacity to translate vision into reality.

—Warren Bennis

The end in mind is to explode your practice. But first *you* must define what that means to *you*! What is your *vision*? What do you want your life to look like in ten years? You must paint this picture in detail first. Success in any aspect of life starts here—a clean, specific picture of where you are going.

Sit down with a yellow legal pad and write out your biggest dreams. Be as extravagant and crazy as possible—no limits, let your mind run wild. In detail, imagine what your life will look like spiritually, physically, and emotionally. Imagine your relationships, marriage, kids, finances, your office volume, collections, vacations, and hobbies. What is your utopia, your deepest desire? When you put your dreams in writing, you wake up your vision. Go for it, and think *big*.

Who in life has accomplished what you desire? Find a group or individual you can model. The mentorship group that catapulted my life was the Dynamic Essentials Conference started by Dr. Sid E. Williams. This is where my vision became reality. Call them up, write them, visit them. Create a relationship that allows you space to learn what it took to get them where they are. Learn what they did right and what they did "wrong." Build off their strengths and what they would have done differently. When given clear advice, don't say, "Yeah but" or "What if…" Just do it. Take action!

A major key to any success is to take *massive action*. Do not overthink every little step. If a voice in your head says, "Do this," and it feels right, *do it*! There is no such thing as a mistake in this action. Don't be overattached to the results, just keep moving forward. Failure begins when you allow the educated mind to override your innate. It is one thing to dream, but we must wake up and work. Master an upper cervical technique. This is where the greatest results and certainty in practice will come. The greatest way to build a practice is referral. The best way to receive referrals is through results. I practice evidence-based chiropractic; our patients get well, and that's evidence. Results speak louder than words, and the answer lies between the atlas! How's your atlas? Hustle! Make relationships, and sell the principle of chiropractic. Communicate how chiropractic will add value to people's lives, and serve them with love. Review your vision daily. Enjoy the journey up your mountain, but know that once you get to the top, there is a bigger mountain somewhere else. So enjoy the journey. Love life, and life will love you back!

Judson Family Chiropractic Mission

We serve as their lighthouse to lead them through the darkness of manipulation and greed. Our intentions, when pure and delivered through a masterful adjustment, release the chains the atlas subluxation bears. Our journey is to live clearly, master our emotions, maintain a state of love, and master our art as chiropractors.

A dream is what makes people love life even when it's painful.

—Theodore Zeldin

PRINCIPLE 18

Evidence of Life
Phil McMaster, DC

• • •

The signs of life are evidence of the intelligence of life.

IT WOULD SEEM LOGICAL TO state what the five signs of life are first in order to help you further understand the significance of the principle in which they are alluded to.

It should be pointed out that these signs of life are commonly accepted as true and accurate in the scientific world and are not a chiropractic creation. They are somewhat self-evident in any cursory observation of living organisms.

FIVE SIGNS OF LIFE
Assimilation (Matter/Energy Exchange)

Assimilation is "the ability of an organism to take into its body food materials selectively and make them a part of itself according to a system or intelligent plan" (*Chiropractic Text Book*, 35). Food, water, oxygen, and information are all actively assimilated from the environment into the organism. Assimilation is self-directed—determined by the needs of the organism. Environmental "assimilants" must be *adapted* (purposefully altered) to be utilized. All matter must be reorganized into the forms adapted to the organism's needs. The information in any force must be converted from destructive to constructive. Information must be translated into meaningful form (understanding).

Elimination (Matter/Energy Exchange)

Elimination is "the ability of an organism to give off waste matters selectively, which an intelligence deems are no longer of use in that structure" (*Chiropractic Text Book*, 35). The waste products of metabolism are selectively and actively expelled back into the environment. Elimination is self-directed—determined by the needs of the organism. Matter and energy are eliminated by the body: metabolic waste matter (CO_2, H_2O, NH_3), excess energy, unassimilated dietary elements, autotoxins (breakdown products), immune system effluvia, and surface epidermal layer. It is a common origin of the perception of *sickness*—nausea, diarrhea, fever, and so on.

Growth (Self-Assembly/Self-Transformation)

Growth is "the ability to expand according to an intelligent plan to mature size" (*Chiropractic Text Book*, 37). The body's innate intelligence uses assimilated energy to assemble matter into the structures and functions of life. Growth is self-directed—influenced by the genetic potentials and environmental "assimilants" but determined by the expression of innate intelligence appropriate for different stages of life:

- Embryology—rapid self-assembly, assimilation vastly exceeding elimination
- Maturation—developmental growth, assimilation exceeding elimination
- Education—informational growth, continuous assimilation/integration of new experiences
- Dynamic equilibrium—self-maintenance, assimilation approximately equaling elimination

Reproduction (Metaunital [Life] Perpetuation)

Reproduction is "the ability of the unit to reproduce something of like kind; the power to perpetuate its own kind" (*Chiropractic Text Book*, 38). Reproduction is "metaunital" (beyond the needs of the organism itself). Cellular reproduction is directed by the organism's needs. Organismic reproduction is directed by the needs of the species. Molecular replication may be the earliest, simplest "sign" of life. Asexual reproduction is fission, cloning, and budding. All are types of the "duplication of form." Sexual (gametal) reproduction also produces a "duplication of form." It produces variation of form through which the "consciousness of life" *can express itself fully.*

Adaptability

Adaptability is the ability a living organism has to respond to all forces that impinge on it, both internal and external, so as to survive as itself. The *ability* to adapt comes from the *innate intelligence* of the organism. The expression of that ability comes from the material organization (structure/function) of the organism. It is often considered the primary sign of life. Adaptability is "the intellectual ability that an organism possesses of responding to all forces which come to it, whether Innate or Universal" (*Chiropractic Text Book*, 36). It is expressed at all levels of living function. Adaptability is a potential (the ability to respond) that must be expressed moment by moment as actual responses (adaptations). Adaptability is intellectual, whereas adaptations are physical.

By definition, a living organism is organized by a specific portion of universal intelligence (the assumed cause of organization of all things) called innate intelligence. *Intelligence* is from the Latin verb *intelligere*, meaning "to perceive, understand." It is perception, discernment, the ability to respond quickly and successfully to a new situation.

There are two levels of "perception" in a living thing:

- What is happening inside me = internal needs
- What is going on around me = external challenges

And there are two levels of "response" in a living thing:

- How I meet my own needs = coordination
- How I respond to the environment = adaptation

Life is self-created, self-directed motion. Life exists "far from equilibrium." Life demonstrates enthalpy. Death allows equilibrium to return. Death "closes the system," creating entropy.

So, simply put, the self-assembly, self-maintenance, self-transformation, species-perpetuating, and self-directed matter or energy exchanges with the environment. All is done successfully with the life's existence being the end result. This *is* evidence of the expression of a living organism's innate intelligence—higher-order interactive processes that characterize life itself.

There is nothing accidental about this. It is intelligence at work!

Signs of Life
Joe Donofrio, DC

• • •

> There is always new life trying to emerge in each of us. Too often, we ignore the signs of resurrection and cling to part of life that have died for us.
>
> —Joan D. Chittister

> One of the first signs of a spirit filled life is enthusiasm.
>
> —A. B. Simpson

Stephenson's textbook discusses the five signs of life as they relate to the living organism. However, I've often thought that those same signs could be used to productively examine a practice to determine if it is a healthy/live practice *or* a vegetative/dead practice.

Let's look at the first sign of life, assimilation. Does your practice have a steady flow of high-quality "food materials," which are absorbed and become a part of the very body of your practice? These foods are more important in their quality rather than their quantity. An overwhelming number of garbage food people will deceptively weaken the practice body while appearing to "grow" it.

The next sign is excretion, the ability to give off waste matter selectively. Does your practice have mechanisms to eliminate the "garbage or toxins" selectively, before the practice organism is poisoned? Is there a specific mechanism to purge the poisoned people who will kill the practice?

You can control much of the assimilation and its quality and the excretion of the toxic by simply dedicating yourself to a complete and extensive orientation. Let every practice member know who you are, what you do and how you do it, what you have, and what they can expect. You will improve the quality of your practice food and eliminate those who will poison your practice. Remember, likes refer likes. A bad pm will duplicate himself over and over.

Next is adaptability. Does the practice have the flexibility to bend but not break as circumstances change? The changes in insurance practices or regulations will surely challenge your ability to function in an "as usual" way, and challenges from the outside may prove to be fatal to some. Have you created a plan for adapting? Or will you just hope for the best?

The degree of adaptability depends entirely upon the skills and desires of the chiropractor. Can you explore new ideas and open yourself to new thinking without altering the basic principles you live by, especially the chiropractic principles? If you cannot bend while holding to principle, you may face the possibility of breaking.

The fourth sign of life is growth. Is the practice a growing, living, vital organism? Did you see more visits and make more money this month than you did this month last year or the year before or the year before that? If you do not grow, you are either static or dying, and neither of these are signs of life. Growth can be measured objectively as in numbers and subjectively as in the depth of chiropractic understanding of yourself and your practice members.

Reproduction is the fifth sign of life. Are you reproducing a clear, logical, inspirational message day after day? How about the quality of your ability to locate, analyze, and correct vertebral subluxations? Remember, you are only as good as your last visit! Has your practice reached the state where quality members are reproducing other quality members?

Your ability to have a practice reaching its potential in aliveness takes work, help from mentors and friends, and constant alignment. Be vigilant, and be truthful with yourself. A practice is always moving toward life or toward death. The choice is yours.

> **Life is but the expression of spirit through matter. To make life manifest requires the union of spirit and body.**
>
> **—D. D. Palmer**

PRINCIPLE 19

Organic Matter
Eric Russell, DC

• • •

The material of the body of a "living thing" is organized matter.

This is a pretty interesting principle when you read the thirty-three principles overall because we are transitioning from an understanding of universal intelligence, as presented in principles 1 through 17, which is in all matter and continually gives to it its properties and actions and thus maintains it in existence, to our discussion of innate intelligence.

If you have been reading the principles in order, you have been watching how universal intelligence gives force to both living (organic) and nonliving (inorganic) matter. This was set up in particular by principles 16 and 18; the concept of how "living things" are different from nonliving is being introduced through a discussion of the unique properties living things have (the five signs of life).

Matter that is not biologically "alive" still expresses intelligence through organization. This organization is the expression of intelligence through matter by way of a connecting force. Living things are also organized and have an intelligence that is constantly on the job for the purpose of optimal adaptation to the body's internal and external environment.

A living body must constantly build up against entropy and the breakdown that comes from being exposed to universal forces. This buildup is not done without intelligence on the job, which guides the adaptive process toward optimal function.

How do you explain this principle to the public?

33

Current estimates show that there are approximately 37.2 trillion cells in the human body. These cells do not come together purely by accident. Cells function in a highly organized way, and we call that cellular intelligence. Cells group together to form tissues and have tissue intelligence. Tissues come together to form organs, and we call that organ intelligence. Organs come together and form systems and function with system intelligence. Finally, systems form you, and we call that body intelligence.

Nothing in the body happens by random chance. Every cell and function of the body is organized, and that organization helps the body adapt and strive for optimal function of the body. That is the intelligence that drives your self-healing and self-regulation and gets your body to perform at its best.

How does this principle apply to the correction of vertebral subluxation and practice?

The body of a living thing is special and is constantly on the job, building up the body as it adapts. The body does this through constant communication from the intelligence that governs self-healing and self-regulation, and that intelligence is called "innate intelligence."

Innate intelligence provides constant direction to all the tissue cells in the body through a communication called the mental impulse. It is like a general in the field who is directing troops. If this communication gets interfered with, the body loses its communication and that is called a vertebral subluxation. A chiropractor who is highly trained in detecting and facilitating the correction of vertebral subluxation will give a very specific input into the spine to improve the biomechanics, remove any nerve interference or disturbances, and help the body better self-heal and self-regulate, so the patient will enjoy a better quality of life!

Can you give some examples of this principle in action?

Living things act completely differently than nonliving things. Let us look at the different systems of the body. As we said earlier, cells organize to form tissues, and tissues come together to form organs. Organs work together to form systems. The human body has eleven different organ systems functioning together for the wonderful human organism that is you.

Think about it. We have the circulatory, digestive, endocrine, excretory (urinary), immune (lymphatic), integumentary, muscular, nervous, reproductive, respiratory, and skeletal systems that work together in your body to help your body perform at its best.

The immune system is a fascinating example. There are two types of immunity, general and specific. General immunity is something that happens when your body recognizes something does not belong. One of the first lines of defense an intelligent body has is to raise the temperature so it can make a very hostile environment for the invader. Next, it creates specific antibodies to combat the antigen it was exposed to. Not only that, but the immunity is "learned" by the body. The body adapts and remembers this antigen and has antibodies ready.

Isn't it amazing just how smart the body is? By being organized, the body works with coordinating and organized parts for the purpose of adaptation. The material of a living thing (you) is organized.

How does this principle apply to life?

These examples demonstrate just how brilliant and intelligent the universe is. All things in the universe are organized, both living and nonliving.

Just recently, I was teaching this concept to a class of freshman chiropractic students. To demonstrate the organization of the universe, I played a short video of Fibonacci numbers in nature. The main point of the video is to show the viewer that nature has a repeating frequency or organization to it. It is often called the golden mean or phi. That ratio is 1:1.618, and it is found almost everywhere in nature, especially when one is looking at plants. The Fibonacci sequence is represented by 1.1.2.3.5.8.13.21.34.55…and you add the last two numbers together to get the next number in the pattern. The golden mean ratio is when you divide the previous number by the last number (especially when you get to the higher numbers).

So the leaves of a plant are usually 3, 5, and 8, or some number in the sequence. The golden mean can be found all over the human body. If you take the difference of your hand, that is usually 1 and your hand and forearm together is 1.618.

33

After I gave the lecture, a student took the time to e-mail me the response that learning the universe is intelligent really blew her mind. She had never thought about it or looked for it, but once she saw it, she could only see organization. Organization implies intelligence, and it is that intelligence that organizes you. It is a great power indeed and does brilliant things without interference.

> **Innate is God within human beings. Innate is good in human beings. Innate cannot be cheated, violated, or tricked. Innate is always waiting, ready to communicate with you, and when innate is in contact, you are in tune with the infinite.**
>
> —B. J. Palmer

The Bigness of Chiropractic
Arno Burnier, DC

● ● ●

The most pathetic person in the world is someone who has sight but no vision.

—Hellen Keller

Get the Big Idea and all else follows.

—B. J. Palmer

THE BIGNESS OF CHIROPRACTIC IS that our philosophy and principles are seeding a new paradigm for life, health, healing, and well-being. It is a paradigm that, in time, will replace the antiquated, mechanistic, crisis-care-and-symptom-suppression medical paradigm of so-called health care. Emergency, life-saving medicine will always be necessary and a salvation to all of those needing it.

Chiropractic has an opportunity at the present time, like never before, to bring forth a new design for living. In essence, the bigness of chiropractic is that it is the "Cousteau Society" of the internal environment of humanity, honoring the sanctity of the human body.

The next step in human evolution, in regard to life, health, and healing, will be to be proactive rather than reactive, to support the healing process rather than to suppress the symptoms, and to promote health

33

rather than to fight disease. This new step means taking care of ourselves, doing something positive for our own being and physiology on a regular basis from conception to transition.

The bigness of chiropractic is the knowledge and understanding of the natural laws that govern life, nature, and human beings, as we are part of life and nature, not separated from it. It is to acknowledge, in a humble way, the bewildering inborn innate intelligence that resides in all beings. It is to stand in awe at the mystery of life and the universe, knowing that we only know and understand but a minuscule fraction of it all. It is to be able to trust the inner wisdom of our being in guiding us, healing us, and sustaining us in health and in sickness.

The bigness of chiropractic is the realization that humanity does not need another therapy. One more therapy will not make a difference, as there are countless new therapies popping up every year, all promising to be the new rising shining star, only to become, over time, a falling star.

It is the realization that what humanity needs is a rudder, a compass, a GPS to live life by and that these honing devices reside within. It is by living from the inner guidance, from the inside out, connected to our own spirit, that we contribute to the evolution of humanity.

The bigness of chiropractic becomes apparent when one reads the books of anatomy, physiology, pathology, biochemistry, and biophysics as spiritual texts, because they reveal, not the knowledge we humans have about these subjects but rather the ingenious mind of the designer, the architect, the inventor of all the parts, organs, and systems of our being.

It is when one realizes that we humans have never discovered or invented anything that did not first exist in nature or within ourselves that the bigness of chiropractic emerges. Indeed, we humans only uncover what already existed long before we were even a thought in our parents' minds.

The bigness of chiropractic is expressed through the loving hands and open hearts of Doctors of Chiropractic who stand in humble awe at the magic and mystery of life and implicitly trust the power of total presence in an innate-to-innate connection, with all the people being served via the chiropractic adjustment.

> **If there can be some paradigm shift
> that you're part of, that's cool.**
>
> —S<small>TEPHEN</small> M<small>ALKMUS</small>

PRINCIPLE 20

Innate Intelligence
Steve Tullius, DC

• • •

A "living thing" has an inborn intelligence within its body, called Innate Intelligence.

THIS STATEMENT REPRESENTS THE ESSENCE of chiropractic's philosophy.

In a single, simple sentence, volumes are told. It shares what the public already knows but often forgets and casts a solid anchor for chiropractors to steady their ship while serving as a compass to define their course and actions.

Chiropractic, like other natural-healing professions, recognizes this inherent, inborn intelligent nature of life and this guiding intelligent force that is constantly striving to produce and express optimal health and function.

When we start with this deep awareness that there is an innate intelligence within the body that orchestrates the processes of life, we approach, address, and assist our patients in a very unique manner.

We see them and the wisdom within their bodies as infinitely intelligent. We understand that their natural birthright is one of abundant health and happiness. We see them as whole and know that if they are not expressing optimal health and function, there must have been some form of interference with that process. We recognize that the intelligence within their body is far greater than the educated intelligence that is a product of it. And we know that our educated mind, while an amazing tool, cannot possibly know what that innate intelligence knows in matters concerning the health, wellness, and organization of the body.

And so with this deep respect, acknowledgment, and understanding, the chiropractor seeks not to stimulate, depress, or alter the body in any way but instead to remove interference with the expression of that innate intelligence so that it may heal, restore, repair, and guide that body throughout a lifetime.

This important distinction between the educated intelligence and innate intelligence of the body means that the chiropractor will never do anything to harm the body. Every effort will be placed instead on releasing and restoring the capacity of the innate intelligence of the individual to express itself at its fullest potential. Because that intelligence is constantly striving to maintain that individual in a state of optimal health and function and would never cause harm to the body, the only possible result of removing interference to its expression is improved health, function, and quality of life.

This principle of recognizing that there is an innate intelligence is a simple yet profound philosophic position that guides all our future actions and is a major reason for the amazing results chiropractic sees.

Explaining this principle to the public is simple, yet chiropractors tend to make it rather difficult and more confusing than it needs to be.

We like to overcomplicate a very simple concept that the majority of the world already understands as part of their core beliefs. Approximately 85 percent of the world believes that the universe is intelligently designed. This means that they already accept and believe that their bodies have an inborn wisdom that guides their healing, repair, growth, and function.

The problem is that they are disconnected from that awareness.

They have this vitalistic belief system as their primary background theory; however, they are living and making choices regarding their health and lives that contradict those beliefs because they are inundated with a message that tells them they are designed to be sick, that symptoms and disease are normal, and that they need an outside pill, potion, or authority figure to heal their bodies from the outside in.

Our job as chiropractors is simply to reconnect people with the awareness they already have.

The key is not doing so in an inside-out manner that hammers in this concept but instead through gentle questioning that helps bring their awareness back in alignment with their core beliefs so that they act congruently with those beliefs. When we are successful in doing so, the patient becomes empowered to make decisions regarding their health and life that are congruent with their beliefs and with the fundamental principles of how life and health operate.

This is one of the beautiful results of sharing this principle and the chiropractic philosophy in general. It reconnects the individual with the awareness of an innate intelligence within his or her own body and with the basic principles of health and life, which allow us to be much more capable and confident in handling life's challenges.

Because this principle of innate intelligence is of such great importance to both the chiropractor and the people we serve, explaining this principle is an essential part of patient education.

This education is part of a greater series of key concepts I call the *patient education formula*. I look at this endeavor as a simple exercises in logic that takes the individual on a linear journey that will make sense or not depending upon the truth of each step along the journey.

To communicate this principle of innate intelligence, I start with a very simple question. I ask individuals, "Do you believe our bodies were designed to be healthy or sick?"

Of course, the majority of people will answer that our bodies are designed to be healthy. Once I have agreement with that important point, I can then move on to principle 17, cause and effect. If optimal health and function is our natural, normal state, then it follows that if we find ourselves in a state of symptoms and disease, that there must have been some cause to remove us from health.

From there, I ask them what the ingredients for health are. All of us know the answer—good nutrition, water, sunshine, rest, and a positive mental attitude.

But what if we were to bake a cake with those ingredients and used them out of order? What if we didn't follow the recipe? This is the piece of the health equation that we have neglected and missed for centuries. We have failed to recognize the intelligent process of life and the necessary communication of that intelligence to organize and use the ingredients for health to produce optimal health, function, and quality of life.

Interference with that process necessarily results in dysfunction and ultimately, if present long enough, greater and greater levels of breakdown and decay.

This concept is so simple yet so incredibly vital for people to understand. Using this baking analogy is a simple way to get this important principle across.

In practice, this principle of innate intelligence is extremely relative to the correction of vertebral subluxations. As previously mentioned, the recognition of an innate intelligence means that the chiropractor is only interested in removing interference to the expression of that intelligence. In chiropractic, we have recognized that vertebral subluxations represent one of the most common interferences with that optimal expression.

Having this awareness means that the chiropractor is not misled or guided by the symptoms the body is expressing but instead uses tools and indicators found useful in determining whether or not vertebral subluxation is present. The chiropractor understands that symptoms can be the very intelligent expression of innate intelligence as healing and repair are occurring, and at other times no symptoms will outwardly present themselves, even though the vertebral subluxation is present. To allow the symptoms to guide one's judgment on the appropriateness of an adjustment or to limit one's being checked for vertebral subluxation is a grave error on the part of the chiropractor and society. Understanding that an innate intelligence exists and its role in the active organization of the body makes it imperative that anyone who values optimal health, function, and quality of life be checked for vertebral subluxation throughout a lifetime.

This principle is not only applicable to health and functioning of the body but also to our everyday lives. When we start with the awareness that life is intelligent and that it is constantly striving for optimal expression, we can reflect on multiple areas of life, such as relationships, politics, economics, and even our own happiness.

Our understanding of the cyclical process of life in general and of this intelligent information exchange in which information is communicated to a desired target, that information is received, intelligent feedback is given, and then that feedback is received in a continuous cycle allows us to simply step back and analyze where interference may be occurring and make the necessary adjustment in our relationships and social systems. This principle can be applied to practically any situation, problem, or process we wish to improve or evolve.

With this principle and the application of it, society could literally transform and evolve on multiple fronts. The cost effectiveness of a salutogenic, or health promotion, health-care strategy that embraced this principle would be astronomical. The decrease in human sickness and suffering and the ability of individuals to express their fullest potential in all areas of their lives, as well as recognize the inherent intelligence and potential of others, would result in a surge in all areas from arts and sciences to politics and international relations. All of this would result in a pinnacle of human achievement never witnessed or even imagined by some.

In chiropractic, we call this the *big idea*. It is all contained in one short sentence: "A 'living thing' has an inborn intelligence within its body, called innate intelligence."

Build a Chiropractic Dynasty

• • •

How does someone know what they don't want if they have never even seen it.

—STEVE JOBS

The empires of the future are the empires of the minds.

—WINSTON CHURCHILL

YOU WANT TO BUILD A dynasty? Then assume everyone wants chiropractic. They just don't know about it. Your job is to introduce as many people as possible to chiropractic and uncover what they already want and need. Be the Steve Jobs of chiropractic.

Everyone uses cell phones and computers and pays a monthly service for Internet, cell usage, cable, electricity, and so on. Why not chiropractic?

People pay to stay connected to their outer world. What we do is keeping them connected in their inner world and to the universal source. Is there anything more valuable than that? Every aspect of the human experience relies on a clear source-brain-body connection.

I believe a major mistake most chiropractors make is they think because a person comes in with a symptom that they need to address that symptom and meet the person where they are at.

Oftentimes, people are motivated to take action because they have a symptom, but there is something deeper. They are subluxated. That does not mean the vertebral subluxation is the cause of their symptom. What it means is the person is subluxated, disconnected from the inner and outer source.

The innate intelligence does not want vertebral subluxations disrupting information and energy flow. So no matter what they tell you is the reason for seeking your care, it goes much deeper. They are in dis-ease, dis*harmony,* discon*nection. No one's inner wisdom wants to live in this state.*

People pay to be connected to their outside world; they will pay to be connected to their inner world beyond symptom relief. You just have to deliver the goods. This is where I see a major disconnect in our profession. Very often, the quality of our craft, which is the location, analysis, and correction of vertebral subluxation is not up to par with what we tell people. And very often, what we tell people is not up to par with the deeper unconscious reasons for seeking our care.

Underpromise and overdeliver.

—Joel Pilskin

PRINCIPLE 21

The Mission of Innate Intelligence
Patty Cosemeli, DC

● ● ●

The mission of innate intelligence is to maintain the material of the body of a "living thing" in active organization.

How do I explain this principle to my patients or the public?
There is an unseen force or intelligence that binds all matter in our universe; it creates organization in our solar system and our galaxy. This force is what is known as universal intelligence in the philosophical realm of chiropractic. We embrace this intelligence and honor it, and we understand that without the sense of balance that is created, our way of life would not be able to exist. We also understand that, that same intelligence or force expresses itself in our human body, and we call it innate intelligence. We have been hearing a great deal more about the term *innate intelligence* both in scientific journals and in everyday language. I've even seen movies where they reference the term in a manner that makes it common sense to understand the existence of such a force.

Innate intelligence simply exists in all living matter; it is the invisible force that connects and balances everything into an organized living system.

Without a single conscious thought, this intelligence or force organizes and keeps our human body functioning and moving in harmony and synchronicity. In other words, we don't have to think about assisting our heart beating or our lungs breathing or any other organ function; it happens because as innate intelligence simply expresses and organizes matter, the body, and all of our systems work in synchronicity with one another through the vast connections made by our brain and nervous system.

When innate intelligence is allowed to express itself to its fullest potential, our ability to adapt to our environment and all of its stresses and challenges becomes facilitated by a harmonious state of being. Matter becomes organized when needed; this is the mission of innate intelligence. The human body cannot exist and function without innate intelligence expressing through it; the premise is to simply help it express.

How does this principle apply to practice and the correction of vertebral subluxation?

The vertebral subluxation is one of the main causes that create imbalance and disharmony in the human body by creating a disconnect in the maximum expression of innate intelligence. The vertebral subluxation creates an obstruction, if you will. Finding and correcting where exactly that obstruction has occurred is the work that is performed by the chiropractor, and then assisting to restore the expression of innate intelligence is what makes chiropractic so unique in the field of health care.

The work is simple, yet profound, because to be able to assist in restoring harmony to a possible chaotic environment is very rewarding. To be able to watch a person go from having dis-harmony in his or her mind and body to healing and being at peace with him- or herself is where the gift of our work is the most valuable.

A chiropractor does not try to suppress any possible symptoms a person may be expressing, as we don't really know what that person may need. But innate intelligence understands and knows exactly what the person with an ailment needs. We are simply the catalyst to the maximum expression of this unforeseen force.

How does this principle apply to life?

Life has an unseen order in which nature or intelligence flows, and although it cannot be seen, it can most definitely be felt. We can call this the order of nature. This is how nature knows exactly how to keep things in an organized rhythm.

We see this at work in how we go through the cycles of the seasons on our planet. There is organization to how the seasons shift from one to the other and how the animals move south or hibernate as the seasons shift. No one has to do anything; it is the intelligence of nature, which has order at its finest.

Can you give some examples of this principle in action?

This principle in action is seen at every single moment in our lives when nature is allowed to express itself and humanity does not interfere with its natural course of action, especially when an injury has occurred to the body.

Let's, for instance, say your hand was cut by a sharp object. You start to feel the burn and pain, and blood starts to ooze out of the wound.

What exactly is going on to repair the damage made to the opening of your skin? How does the right amount of cellular activity start mending your cut? How does the right amount of blood start to be pumped, the right amount of coagulants and enzymes produced? Why does swelling occur to protect the area from further harm so quickly? The answer lies in the operating system the body automatically has in place, called the innate intelligence.

There is no mystery in this unseen force. We see its magnetic force every single day, and the moment we acknowledge its existence, our world will innately find a path of least resistance.

The key to growth is the introduction to higher dimensions of consciousness into our awareness.

Present-Time Consciousness

• • •

Do not dwell in the past. Do not dream of the future.
Concentrate the mind on the present moment.

—Buddhist saying

When you are here and now, sitting totally,
not jumping ahead, the miracle has happened.
To be in the moment is the miracle.

—Osho

According to Albert Einstein, the *"line between past, present, and future is actually an illusion."* One of the keys to a high-volume subluxation-centered practice is present-time consciousness. Present-time consciousness is when you are fully present, 100 percent in the moment with your mind, body, and spirit. In this space there is no thought of anything else but the person who is in front of you. This is where the magic takes place in practice.

I have spoken to hundreds of high-volume practitioners, and the conclusion is the same. When you are flowing in present-time consciousness and seeing person after person, time becomes an illusion. There have been days in which I saw 50 people in five hours, and people waited, and it felt like I saw 200 people because I *was not fully present. Other days, I saw 125 in five hours, no one waited, and I felt like I saw 50 because I was 100 percent fully in the moment.*

In this place of present-time consciousness, your educated mind has no time to mess with your intuition. This is when you truly enter into the "zone" athletes describe.

Once we did an experiment in our practice and I had the CA ask people how long people thought they were with me. Most said fifteen to twenty minutes, yet they had been in with me two to four minutes maximum. In present-time consciousness, time becomes warped. Most people never experience this state in their lives. In this state, something powerful takes place between you and the person you are serving that cannot be explained in the mechanical world.

> **I have realized that the past and future are real illusions, that they exist in the present, which is what there is and all there is.**
>
> **—Alan W. Watts**

PRINCIPLE 22

The Amount of Innate Intelligence
Gregory A. Stetzel, DC, and Kim R. Stetzel, DC

● ● ●

There is 100 percent of innate intelligence in every "living thing," the requisite amount, proportional to its organization.

MOST CHIROPRACTORS TAKE PRINCIPLE 22 for granted, as it seems a given, based on our philosophical underpinnings that innate intelligence is present in every living thing and that it would be present at 100 percent and equivalent to the needs of the organism to sustain and maintain life. It just makes sense. But how do we incorporate this philosophical tenet into a discussion that can make it a reality for the average person in a way that helps him or her to better understand his or her body and the importance of the location, analysis, and correction of vertebral subluxation?

If innate intelligence is 100 percent present in 100 percent of the cells of an organism—in our case, the human body—then how does the presence or absence of vertebral subluxation affect the life function of that organism? Based upon our understanding of the chiropractic philosophy of life and the thirty-three principles as delineated by Stephenson, innate intelligence cannot be reduced or enhanced and is always 100 percent. Therefore, the presence of vertebral subluxation does not negatively impact the amount of innate intelligence present within the body, and the correction or removal of the vertebral subluxation does not positively impact the amount of innate intelligence present within the body. Innate intelligence remains at 100 percent in each of the cells and in the body collectively.

If what we do as chiropractors in the location, analysis, and correction of the vertebral subluxation does not directly impact innate intelligence with regard to its presence, how does this principle affect the way we practice our art, apply our philosophy, or guide our science in the attempt to better understand the impact of chiropractic care on the body and its expression of life?

THE LAYPERSON

The average person has long been disassociated from any understanding of the inner workings of the body or the complexities of how the components interrelate to create and maintain their existence. People have been inundated with the "outside-in" fallacies of educated intelligence—so much so, that the concept of a perfect, internal intelligence present and in charge from conception to the beginnings of a new life and every moment thereafter is foreign. They have no frame of reference from which to base an understanding of an innate intelligence as the foundation of their existence because they have been taught from their earliest memories that their bodies are inherently incapable of surviving without the external intervention of an educated overseer.

People are finally drawn into a chiropractic office, either by a loss of faith in a health-care model that ignores the internal power of the body to heal, because they think chiropractic is some form of outside-in therapy, or because they have tried everything else and chiropractic is just the next treatment method on the list. They then must be introduced to the possibilities that become available with the understanding that the internal wisdom that is inherent within them knows what to do to restore function and life to the cells, tissues, organs, and systems that are ultimately controlled by their innate intelligence. They must be empowered to see, perhaps for the very first time, that they are uniquely and inherently *capable* of healing from within, provided communication and transmission of their internal, inborn wisdom that is their innate intelligence is restored. They must be led to understand that their body has 100 percent innate intelligence present within each of its cells. The final concept to convey

33

is that the intelligence that created them and grew them from two tiny cells orchestrated and directed the development of every tissue, organ, and system that they need to survive and continues to provide the information needed to heal and recreate those tissues, organs, and systems necessary for them to sustain life and thrive from conception to their last breath.

With a basic understanding of the complexities of the inner workings of the body and the incredible control and coordination that is made possible by the 100 percent presence of innate intelligence, chiropractic patients are empowered to place their faith in their own body's healing ability, provided there is no interference with the coordination of their innate intelligence. They are less beholden to the educated interventions of conventional health care and able to choose their own path to healing, placing their faith in their body's natural abilities.

The Chiropractor

For a chiropractor, steeped in the philosophical concepts of the thirty-three principles and the teachings of D. D. and B. J. Palmer, the development and acceptance of principle 22 lays the foundation for much of the practical application of the chiropractic art and science that reconnects practice members with their potential. Knowing and accepting that innate intelligence is 100 percent present and in the requisite amount required by the cells, tissues, organs, and systems of the body to maintain organization, and thus life, it becomes possible to realize that the purpose of the chiropractor in assisting the life within the patient's body is only to remove interference with its perfect expression of innate intelligence—nothing more, nothing less, nothing else.

It is impossible for the chiropractor, by way of a chiropractic adjustment or the administration of any other form of treatment or modality, to add or detract from the amount of innate intelligence in the body. The chiropractor's only purpose is to remove interference with the expression of the body's innate intelligence and then to allow that intelligence to perform its function free of interference. Used as the filter for everything that is done in the chiropractic practice, this understanding negates the need for utilization of any technique, modality, or procedure that does not specifically address or satisfy this purpose. Additionally, it would be to the benefit of the chiropractor and the chiropractic client to incorporate any and all techniques that effectively remove interference with the complete expression of the body's innate intelligence and optimization of the life of the patient by facilitating in the correction or reduction of the vertebral subluxation. In this sense, the discussion of technique and procedures becomes moot when utilization shifts to fulfillment of purpose.

A doctor-patient relationship based upon the body's inherent ability to care for itself free of interference places the chiropractor more in the role of facilitator than corrector. Many within the chiropractic profession have argued that the chiropractic adjustment does not correct anything and that the purpose of an adjustment is to assist the body in restoring normal function through the removal of interference with the free flow of the mental impulse. When we place full faith in the body's innate intelligence and its inherent wisdom being in place 100 percent at all times, it becomes increasingly reasonable to assume that the body does not need an intervention to produce a higher expression of itself given an appropriate amount of time and resources. The body "knows" what it needs and will utilize its innate intelligence to find or create it.

In essence, the chiropractic adjustment is a product of educated intelligence creating an educated force to stimulate an innate response within the body that will accelerate its adaptation to an educationally perceived problem. It is the hope and intent of the chiropractor in the administration of the chiropractic adjustment that the body will accept and utilize that force to its ultimate benefit. And if innate intelligence is 100 percent present in 100 percent of the cells, organs, tissues, and systems, the removal of interference in the communication between those cells should produce a 100 percent expression of their intelligence.

IN LIFE
In the understanding and acceptance of the thirty-three principles and principle 22 in particular, we have the opportunity to accept that our

33

bodies have the ability to care for themselves. Just as chiropractic patients must learn to accept this premise as the basis of their health, well-being, and existence, the chiropractor must be equally steeped in the acceptance of this premise on a personal level. If chiropractors are unable or unwilling to accept that their own bodies are under the absolute control and coordination of a 100 percent present expression of innate intelligence, then they will not be able to translate that message to their patients with any degree of certainty and will surely slip progressively into allopathy.

Void of the thirty-three principles of life, a person cannot *be* a chiroprac*tor* and cannot fully live the chiropractic lifestyle. Embracing principle 22 is paramount to the chiropractor being able to live as the embodiment of the chiropractic philosophy.

Success in Practice
Thomas Waller, DC

● ● ●

Integrity means congruence. Words and behavior match.

—Nathaniel Branden

Happiness is when what you think, what you say, and what you do are in harmony.

—Mahatma Gandhi

When I think about success in practice and what advice, tips, and values I can pass on to the reader, I am cautious to state with full confidence that my tip will work for everyone. However, when I think further about the question as to what readers are looking for, I know the first question they must ask themselves is "What is success for me?"

With so many possible answers to this question and so many styles of practice, I have come to the conclusion that the only way to succeed in practice is to remain congruent and the only way to be fulfilled in practice is to continue growing. So what does this mean?

Congruency is the state where all your actions are in agreement and alignment with how you feel emotionally about the action. For example, taking the advice of coaches and "experts" may be of benefit, but if they are asking you to do something that innately does not feel comfortable, then the fruits of your labor will be short lived. Whereas if your efforts and actions are comfortable and in agreement with your thoughts and talents, the reward will be greater.

Let me give an example. For me, public speaking is easy. I talk to groups in my community on a weekly basis and travel to audiences around Europe regularly. It is what I am good at and what I am conformable with, so much so that I have built my practice from public talks. However, if I were to tell you that the best way to grow a successful clinic is through talks, I would be lying, for the simple reason that for the person afraid of talking, it would not be. However, if your talents and comfort lie in writing, then write and publish. If you are good at speaking one on one at health screenings, then this is the key!

I hope I make this point clear. While you may be searching for the golden ticket to grow a successful practice in terms of a specific action or strategy, know that the golden ticket lies within you and that the quickest, most enjoyable, and most sustainable way to grow and maintain success in practice is to be congruent.

Growth is the key to fulfillment. Many chiropractors set up practice and initially thrive. They become busy but are soon bored and unfulfilled. This is the danger to not sustaining practice, falling short, and having to start again. I believe that the key to maintaining your success in practice is to constantly be growing. Now this does not always mean in terms of the numbers of patients you serve. It is in all aspects. Should you get comfortable in your technique, dare to grow or learn something new. If you prefer to stay with a technique, then learn to teach it and grow into a space that you are not comfortable in. Allow your team to expand and grow also. If you create a bigger vision for yourself and your team, the only way to achieve it will be through growth, and this aspect of growth will keep you fulfilled.

Growth and congruency will allow you to build the practice of your dreams to the level of success that you have set for yourself. You have huge potential to affect many people; don't let others' agendas or ideas cloud that.

Your chiropractic practice is yours to own. Your impact on this world in the time that you have is yours to determine. Spend time on self-inspection, realize what congruent means to you, and figure out how you can push yourself to grow. This is my key to a successful practice and a successful life.

Trust is congruence between what you say and what you do.

—**Peter Drucker**

PRINCIPLE 23

The Function of Innate Intelligence
Simon Senzon

● ● ●

The function of innate intelligence is to adapt universal forces and matter for use in the body, so that all parts of the body will have coordinated action for mutual benefit.

Rocks, Water, and Life
How is life different from rocks and water? That is a basic question at the heart of chiropractic. The original chiropractors wanted to understand not just how the chiropractic adjustment worked but also how life was different from everything else, like rocks and water, in order to understand how the body is able to heal itself and organize itself.

Let's start with rocks. There are many different types of rocks, but they all have at least two basic attributes, such as they fall apart over time and you can throw them. All rocks fall to pieces. That is the case with anything that is not alive. This seems simple enough to understand. It becomes important when we consider the uniqueness of life. Life creates itself, grows, reproduces, self-organizes, and heals. Rocks don't.

Also, you can throw rocks! Perhaps you can't throw the really big ones like boulders and asteroids, but they all follow the same rules. Once a rock is projected into space (thrown), it continues on course until it hits something, perhaps bounces, and then comes to a stop. We can even calculate (using math and the laws of physics) how far a rock will fly if we throw it. For example, if you know how heavy it is and how hard you throw, you can get a pretty good prediction about where it will land.

Again, life is very different. Imagine throwing a living thing like a bird? You just can't predict what will happen next because it is alive. Living systems are too complex for such a calculation. Life is just too messy to figure out so precisely. The bird might die of fright, or it might take flight. It might lay an egg, or it might attack. The mystery of life is that each new moment is unique and creative.

We might also understand water in similar ways. If we freeze it, the chemical bonds change so that it hardens into ice and crystallizes. If we heat it up, we get steam. Life is like the water because it exists in a transition zone between liquid and crystal. Some have even suggested that our bodies are liquid crystals because of our orderly form. And yet life is very different than water.

For example, if water goes down the drain in the bathtub, it spontaneously merges into a whirlpool. As long as water keeps flowing through that new and emergent structure (the whirlpool), the structure will maintain itself. As soon as the flow stops or the drain gets plugged, the water goes flat.

Our bodies are not very different from this because we take in energy in the form of food, water, and oxygen and use it to power our body's organization. One scientist has even suggested that living systems are complex metabolic whirlpools. That means that as long as we continue to metabolize (digest the energy), our bodies naturally self-organize. Like the whirlpool going down the drain, if we cut off the energy coming in (stop eating or breathing), we die. But unlike the whirlpool, living systems create their own parts! The uniqueness of this process is what the early chiropractors were talking about.

One of the first things that chiropractors figured out was that the body constantly attempts to adapt to the environment. We generally adapt pretty well. We deal with the physical, chemical, emotional, mental, and spiritual stresses as part of normal living. The challenge comes when the body or mind gets knocked out of balance or is forced to deal with more input than it can effectively handle.

One important way the body fails to adapt is when such forces lead to an interference with the body's ability to adapt and thus effectively

33

self-organize. This whole process was summed up by an early chiropractor long ago in a series of principles. One of the principles really captures just how life is different from rocks and water. He wrote, "The function of Innate Intelligence is to adapt universal forces and matter for use in the body, so that all parts of the body will have coordinated action for mutual benefit."

The main idea here is that the body's natural self-healing and self-organizing functions are coordinated by its inborn intelligence. That intelligence functions over the nervous system and coordinates the actions, which are the very functions of being alive.

The universal forces are any input from outside of the body, whether it is normal and natural forces like eating and breathing or stressors like physical, chemical, emotional, mental, and spiritual challenges. If the body cannot fully adapt to one of these, a cascade of incoordination might develop, especially if the expression of this intelligence is interfered with.

The process of adaption within the body is guided by an inherent and inborn intelligence often referred to as innate intelligence. The function of this intelligence is to adapt universal forces and matter for use in the body for coordinated action. This leads to the benefit of healthy function and ultimately the expression of the intelligence.

Your internal GPS

• • •

The master maker of the human body did not create you and then run off and leave you masterless. He stayed on the job as innate, as the fellow within, as nerve transmission controlling every function of life, as spirit from above-down-inside-out, expressing, creating, exploring, directing you in every field and phase of experience so that your home is truly the world and the world is your home.

—B. J. Palmer

I believe based on experience, philosophy and science that our bodies are equipped with an internal guidance system of such an immense magnitude that we have not even begun to realize its profound possibilities.

The HeartMath Institute is a scientific institute designed to study the heart as an energetic system (www.heartmath.org). One of their studies regarding the heart's intuitive abilities is mind blowing. They showed images of beauty, such as majestic nature scenes, and fear-inducing images, such as venomous snakes, to people on a computer screen. The people being tested were hooked up to heart, brain, and body-function monitors. The results were fascinating. Before the people even saw the pictures, their hearts started to respond physiologically. Then once *the pictures appeared, the physiological response went to the brain and then back to the entire body.*

The results of this study are profound. The researchers concluded that the heart has the power to perceive things before they even take place. Not only that, but it responds first and then the brain and rest of body. This is amazing because part of our inner guidance system relies on information flowing from the heart as an energetic system to the brain and back to the body as this study has shown.

Hence, logic would conclude that a vertebral subluxation can cause distortion in our ability to perceive our internal and external world on all levels because of the way it interferes with our nueral pathways. Thus, clearing vertebral subluxations would enable us to have more clarity, precision and connection on an intuitive and innate level. This is something I have observed and experienced over and over in my own life and practice of twenty years and in my opinion is one of chiropractics greatest benefits.

> **I feel there are two people inside of me—me and my intuition. If I go against her, she'll screw me every time, and if I follow her, we get along quite nicely.**
>
> —Kim Basinger

PRINCIPLE 24

The Limits of Adaptation
Peter J. Kevorkian, DC

● ● ●

Innate intelligence adapts forces and matter for the body as long as it can do so without breaking a universal law. Innate intelligence is also limited by the limitations of matter.

INNATE INTELLIGENCE ASSEMBLES FORCES FOR constructive purposes. Its goal is to keep the matter in which it resides unique. It strives to hold in integrity matter for optimal organization and reorganization. The innate intelligence must function under the laws and limitations of the physical universe, whether they are known or unknown.

For example, the hand is a portion of the body that the innate intelligence integrates within the physiology. If a person took a machete and forcefully directed it at the wrist, the matter of the body could not resist that force, nor could it integrate that force into the body, and the machete would slice off the hand. This is a crude demonstration of the limitations of the matter of the body. All matter has physical properties and characteristics by design. The limitation of matter is determined by that design.

Simply stated, the limitation of matter is the framework within which all matter behaves. The molecules, atoms, and tissues have physical laws governing how they exist and behave. They cannot be any different than their natural design.

A vertebral subluxation happens when the body is unable to integrate and process a force to which the body is subjected. It is a misalignment of spinal bones and a related irritation and obstruction of the nerves.

33

Vertebral subluxations occur as a limitation of matter. When the body is subjected to a force that it cannot fully adapt or integrate, the spine will subluxate. That subluxation will allow less adaptability of the body for its integrity and well-being.

Often, people seek chiropractic care to find a resolution to a health problem or body concern. As much as the objective of chiropractic care is to locate and remove nerve interference (vertebral subluxation), the resolve that many have found to diseases and problems of all sorts is due to a healthier and stronger body and not a specific "treatment." Some chiropractors articulate that when a health problem does not resolve, it is due to the limitation of matter. Although that is an accurate statement, it is important to realize that the body is always better off with good nerve energy than with reduced nerve energy. Subluxation correction is always a benefit to the body.

If we step back and consider all of the principles, principle 24 must fit within the deductive process. The major premise honors the intelligent organizational property of the universe. If we accept the fact that the entire universe is organized and that there is a reason for everything, whether or not we know what that reason is, then there is a reason why there may be limits to matter. Recognizing this, when we do encounter limitations to matter, there is a reason and purpose. Behind that reason is an understanding that the effects of that limitation are of intelligent design. As much as some of the experiences of the body are not pleasant, there is a reason for every condition, pathology, or disease process. If the limitations of matter keep the body in a pathological state, there is intelligent design for that to occur. We may never understand the "why."

Within life, it is healthy for us to realize that there are limitations. We must learn to understand these limitations and how they affect our lives. Limitations existing in physical matter are sometimes easier to witness than those of the mind. Both can adversely affect us or may serve to empower us. It is facing limitations that often opens opportunity and creates adaptability.

We will face limitations of matter in physical recovery, disease, physical endurance, performance, and life experiences. The first step is to recognize the limitation. The second is to continue to do things that you know can only benefit the system regardless of the limitation: eat well, maintain loving relationships, keep moving, be mindful, get real rest, deal with stressors, and keep good nerve supply. The third step is to allow life to do what life needs to do. Surrender into the fact that there is a plan to the universe and we are all a part of that plan.

Relationship and Connection

• • •

Personal revolution does and can have global effects. As we go so goes the world, for the world is us. The revolution that will save the world is ultimately a personal one.

—Marianne Williamson

Love one another, but make not a bond of love: let it rather be a moving sea between the shores of your souls.

—Khalil Gibran

Practices are built on relationships. You want to build a large dream practice? Build large dream relationships. Want more kids? Then show genuine love and interest to the parents and get to know all about their children. Want more referrals? Get to know about people's friends. Any marketing company or sales expert will agree 100 percent that the best publicity is word of mouth. Word of mouth is not only powerful and effective, but it also costs much less.

So how do we tap into this omnipotent rule in marketing? We build relationships, serve people with love, build trust, and give them exceptional chiropractic service each and every visit.

I recently saw a special about a top chef in Indonesia. His restaurant had a one-year waiting list, and people often returned year after year from afar. He had no menu. He decided what you would be eating that evening. His philosophy was simple. Give people a dining experience that can never ever be matched in their entire lives. He said, "Once people eat my food and experience my restaurant, they will never be able to experience food in the same way; nothing will come close."

This is how we have to set up and enter into our practices each day. We strive to create the exceptional chiropractic experience while building powerful relationships with the people we serve.

Five Points of Action

1. *Ask about their family in detail, for example, "Marcos, tell me about your kids? How old are they? What are their names? What do they like to do?"*
2. *Ask about their friends. "Marcos, tell about some of your friends? What do you all like to do for fun? What do you all have in common?"*
   I always then bring the conversation at some point back to chiropractic because I truly love people enough to want to serve them all with my gift of chiropractic. I dol this is in precise, on-point, quick communications.
3. *Use voice mail and whats app messages. After any new person begins care in my practice or a client changes levels of care or brings his or her children, I leave a personalized voice-mail message. The following is an example.*
   "Pablo, this is David Serio, your chiropractor. I want to thank you for the opportunity to introduce you to chiropractic. I want you to know I am here to serve you and your family and friends. Thank you once again. I will see you on Thursday at six for your second visit. Have a great day!"
   This implies that Pablo now has himself a chiropractor, that I care about and love him as a human being, that I am grateful to serve him, and that I want to serve his friends and family—all in a thirty-second-or-less message!
4. *Write gratitude letters. Each day in our practice, the CA and the chiropractor write one to three handwritten letters of gratitude to people, which they receive on their following visit. Here are two samples:*

Maria. Thank you for being regular with your care this week. I was able to give you the very best care possible because of your consistency.

—D<small>AVID</small>

Simon. Thank you for showing up for your visits on time and with consistency. I so appreciate you.

—M<small>ONICA, CHIROPRACTIC ASSISTANT</small>

This exercise keeps the chiropractor and staff focused on gratitude, which is the key to abundance; focuses on what people are doing right in our practice rather than scolding them for not doing things the way we think they should; shows them in the written word we care about them; and shows that we pay attention.

5. Stay positive. People have enough negative energy, words, interactions, and situations that they encounter each day. They crave positive vibes. We make it a rule in our practice that once they walk through our door, if they have nothing inspiring or positive to say, be in silence. We have created such a positive environment that they do not want to miss one visit or one week without coming into our practice.

We are drowning in information while starving for wisdom. The world henceforth will be run by synthesizers, people able to put together the right information at the right time, think critically about it, and make important choices wisely.

—E. O. W<small>ILSON</small>

PRINCIPLE 25

The Character of Innate Forces
Sharon Gorman, DC

• • •

**The forces of innate intelligence never
injure or destroy the structures in which they work.**

When I was in chiropractic school, I learned that there is nothing more scientific than chiropractic. If we were trying to figure the body out from the outside in, like medical doctors, we would need to be discovering more about the body every year. That is why the medics are always changing and discovering new drugs to prescribe and altering their surgical procedures and protocols. When using their education, there is always more to discover. The reason that I say that nothing is more scientific than chiropractic is because I know that if a person has a subluxation, there is never an instant that the body is better off not having that subluxation cleared. We might alter our technique, but the bottom line is that the innate does the healing and knows a lot more than we do, so if we clear the interference, the power that made the body can heal the body. Of course, there are limitations of matter and sometimes medical intervention might be necessary if the tissue cells are already destroyed and the body needs more time to repair itself, but whether the symptoms will ever go away or the tissue will ever heal, the person is still better off having the subluxations removed because they always interfere with the expression of innate intelligence.

The innate intelligence that exists in our body is the difference between life and death. The body can't heal if it is not alive. As we clear people's nervous systems, the organization that occurs as a by-product of the life-force can function. Without that intelligence, the body decays. I often tell my people, "Rigor mortis starts in your spine." If innate can't express itself in our bodies, then we start to decay.

I spend a lot of time explaining this concept to patients because I specialize in lifetime family care. I want to encourage my people to keep their nervous systems clear so they can best adapt to the environment and the stresses of life. I often tell my people that I am working with the body that they take to the gym, not the body they take to the drugstore, meaning that each adjustment builds on the last, and the goal is to create a system that functions in the best possible way by restoring proper function. I ask them to make a commitment to their life and health and to invest not only in the present but in their future by being committed to caring for their nervous system on a regular basis throughout their lives.

I also explain that symptoms aren't necessarily bad, but they are your body's way of communicating with you. Our goal should not be simply to remove their symptoms—just like the goal of having a fire alarm is not to silence it even if there is a fire.

From the minute they walk into my office, they can tell that my office isn't the office of a traditional doctor. I take pride in that. The walls speak to them along with videos explaining the processes of the office and what they can expect from us during care. I do a patient-education class every week, and I explain to them where healing comes from and the importance of keeping their "power on."

I think that we need to continue to work on having the term *subluxation* be a household one. We need to make it real for people. When people find out they have cancer, they get how serious a health issue it is. I am working on having people understand that the subluxation is just as deadly and way deadlier than tooth decay. People wouldn't think of waiting for a toothache before getting a dental checkup. Since subluxations are often painless, especially in the early stages, the only way they would know if they are subluxated is if they get their spine checked.

This principle relates to life and especially the life of a chiropractor. I know that when I give an adjustment, the force that I put into the person's spine clears it of interference so the person can heal. I don't heal the patient. I help the body by decreasing interference. In my life, I work on functioning by being in the flow of that intelligence and continually listening to the voice within. I try to tap into that same wisdom that knows that the newborn child should go to the breast or that intelligence that heals a paper cut on your finger even if you forget to put a bandage on it. I meditate daily, and I try to line up my life with *life* and to be of most use to my fellow humans by being an example of living an "innate life."

When talking to my people during their adjustments, I work on sharing with them the chiropractic principles, including this one. The principle is what keeps them in the office. Most people come to the office because they have pain, but if I felt my job was to remove their pain, their care in my office would be limited. Let's face it; when people come into my office, they are going to feel better, feel worse, or feel the same. In any of these scenarios, they would have no reason to remain under care. It's the principle that makes sense and keeps them in the practice. It keeps me getting my spine checked even though I've been having my spine checked for forty-five years.

So here is one of my favorite examples. I ask people why not everyone has hay fever during "allergy season." Often in a particular area of the world, some people get hay fever, and some don't. The people who get hay fever don't have the ability to adapt to the outside environment as well as people who don't express symptoms of hay fever. Their body heals better. I often tell people that their adjustment might not make them feel better, but it will make them heal better. They heal better because of this principle. Innate intelligence never injures or destroys the structures in which they work.

I also tell them about Dr. Sid. He would drop his keys during his lecture, and naturally, they would fall down. He would say, "Just like gravity, chiropractic works every time." There is never a case in which someone is better off subluxated. The body always works better if the innate can be expressed—every time.

Each time I lay my hands on someone, I know that I am doing good for that person no matter what happens with his or her symptoms, and I also know that not only am I doing a service for him or her, but I am also

33

doing a service for his or her unborn children because as the body can express life, they are going to get closer to being able to live their genetic potential.

When I talk with chiropractic students (which I often have the privilege to do), I tell them that if we had to sum up the product that we are bringing to the world in one word, the word would be *aliveness*. We turn on life in people. I can't think of a worthier product. I've been doing this work for over thirty years, and I'm just getting started. I'm more excited to be a chiropractor today than I was the day I graduated from school. Not too many professionals can say that.

Futurism and Thriving

• • •

The measure of who we are is what we do with what we have.

—Vince Lombardi

Surviving is important. Thriving is elegant.

—Maya Angelou

THRIVE: (MERRIAM-WEBSTER) TO FLOURISH

I see chiropractic as a technology for human thriving, included in this would be health, of course, which is one major aspect of a human thriving. There are literally thousands of technologies to help us thrive as human beings, many ancient and many new ones coming to life daily—technologies, such as NLP, yoga, meditation, nutrition, mindfulness, and Reik are just some of examples. In my opinion, chiropractic goes above and beyond any and all of the other human-enhancement technologies, because on a scientific level, we are working with the physical and physiological center of the human body. The central nervous system is the master controller and coordinator of every cell, tissue, and organ.

The neural-spinal system is the energetic and mechanical center that affects everything you are doing in your life and enables you to adapt and experience life at the highest level. No matter what else you do, you cannot get the most out of any experience in life if your neural-spinal system has a vertebral subluxation.

These are a few of the reasons why the number-one coach in the world, Anthony Robbins, utilizes chiropractic on a regular basis. He gets the importance of a clear nervous system for life and in enhancing our ability to thrive and adapt. Tony Robbins repeatedly states the importance of being healthy from the inside out if we are to thrive as human beings. Chiropractic is at the forefront of this human-potential movement.

There are more and more people seeking answers to living a long, prosperous, healthy, vital, and vibrant life. In fact, leading futurists say that one of the major businesses of the future will be anything that focuses on helping us live longer and add quality to our lives. The current reality is that consumers are already spending billions and billions of dollars per year in the search for the fountain of youth.

These are just some of the reasons why chiropractic has never been better positioned to make maximum impact. We provide a major solution for people in their search for a more vibrant, vital life. Chiropractic also provides a major solution to our increasingly emotionally and physically toxic, polluted environment because a nervous system free of vertebral subluxation enables us to adapt to the best of our ability to our environment.

**In order to thrive, connect to and engage to
what is Life-Generating and avoid or prevent
what is Life-Depleting in any way you can.**

—AUTHOR UNKNOWN

PRINCIPLE 26

Comparison of Universal and Innate Forces
Richard John Grostic, DC

• • •

In order to carry on the universal cycle of life, universal forces are destructive and innate forces constructive, as regards structural matter.

THE COMBINED THIRTY-THREE PRINCIPLES CONCEPTUALLY provide for a philosophy that offers a basic understanding of life itself. The principles embody a chiropractic adjustment and the restorative role the adjustment plays in health and disease.

The early writings of chiropractic pioneers gravitated toward a more pantheistic viewpoint, congruent with and adaptable to many, if not all, theological and ideological beliefs. Chiropractic philosopher R. W. Stephenson published the *Chiropractic Text Book* in 1937. His writings included the thirty-three principles, adopted by many leaders in the profession and accepted as an educational construct offering guidance and understanding for the chiropractic profession. The principles directly and indirectly offer a plausible foundation from which a profession was born and since has served to change countless lives.

In order to carry on the universal cycle of life, universal forces are destructive and innate forces constructive, as regards structural matter.

Before one can begin to fully comprehend principle 26, it is best to gain an understanding of its components, beginning with knowing that universal intelligence forces are part of an all-encompassing and omnipotent totality of all existence. Universal intelligence is what animates you and everything around you. Ponder the things surrounding you, and understandably, you recognize that everything is made of atoms. Atoms have an infinite energy with forces that can form bonds or repel one another. This energy that binds or repels is an example of universal intelligence (force) and is found quite literally everywhere you can imagine. Universal intelligence provides an intrinsic tendency for things to organize and coalesce, intricately interwoven into various forms of matter. Universal intelligence is a miracle in and of itself, but something even bigger is at play when you combine and arrange these atoms.

Think for a moment about the following six atoms: carbon, oxygen, hydrogen, nitrogen, calcium, and phosphorous. These atoms are combined in various forms to comprise almost 99 percent of your body. Now, simply add another five atoms: magnesium, potassium, sodium, chlorine, and sulfur. All eleven of these basic ingredients are required for life and make up close to 100 percent of your body's composition. These ingredients, guided by universal intelligence, are *you* and can be found in and around *you*. Something miraculous differentiates the ingredients found within you from those around you. Within you is a force, a life-force known by many as innate intelligence. This inborn intelligence gives to those ingredients from which you are composed, organizing them into a seemingly miraculous order for one specific purpose. This purpose, the miracle, is your life!

A universal cycle of life cannot be denied, as it pertains to all living organisms. Take for example one small acorn or oak nut, a single seed housed in a tough, leathery shell with a small cap. This one small acorn has housed within it the potential to become one of many majestic and enormous oak trees. On average, it takes twenty to thirty years for a mature oak tree to produce the same acorns from whence it came. An oak tree has the potential to live a hundred years or more, dependent on its innate ability to overcome. The oak tree, while a magnificent sight to behold, is weathered and endures much throughout its life, and it ultimately returns to the soil the very atoms from which it came.

A universal life cycle implies a series of changes in form that an organism undergoes while ultimately returning to its starting point components.

In the Bible, we read, "In the sweat of thy face shalt thou eat bread, till thou return unto the ground; for out of it wast thou taken: for dust thou art, and unto dust shalt thou return" (Gen. 3:19 KJV). Should innate forces be withdrawn from any living organism, it will ultimately revert to the elemental state from which it came. Destructive forces, a desire to take back what has been loaned to the innate, can be summed up as mortality. The universal cycle of life, seen historically and evidenced from that of a mere acorn to the many oak trees that offer life, perpetuated through the production of new acorns, giving rise to new trees.

Similar to the small acorn, you came from a lineage of generations, all borrowing from universal intelligence elements that when combined with the innate offer life, a mortal life. Upon this earth, you are a living organism composed of materials provided for you by universal intelligence. It should be clear that the function of the innate is to package the materials provided by universal intelligence so life can emanate from your being. Your body experiences a multitude of cycles, such as sleep, breathing, and body temperature. Certainly you don't sit around telling your heart to beat or have to remind yourself to breathe. These are just a few simple and basic examples of your very own salubrious innate intelligence. Innate intelligence seeks balance and harmony within your body. Chiropractors facilitate this balance by removing interference and restoring balance. Innate intelligence has an all-important job and the seemingly simple task of keeping you alive. It encompasses a myriad of complicated processes simultaneously orchestrated to give *you* life.

From your conception, your innate design began to lay a foundation. Cells divided and multiplied, specializing in purpose, setting in motion the creation of a special communication network. Beginning with your brain, the location where your innate intelligence takes up residence and sets up as a primary control center. The human brain is the one mathematically absolute place from which the innate governs the body and coordinates its actions. By design, your brain regulates, controls, and manages your body. Your brain is housed within a protective bone structure called your skull. Your brain gives rise to a spinal cord with a large network of nearly forty-five miles of nerves running throughout your body. Your spinal cord

33

is protected by more than twenty-four articulating bones, providing a passage for communication lines between your brain and body. Innate intelligence uses this network of nerves to self-regulate and maintain a balance of the materials provided by universal intelligence. Nerve supply or innate communication between your brain and body is addressed by chiropractors, providing for an optimal expression of your innate intelligence.

In summary, universal forces are destructive as a means of completing the universal cycles of life by defining the mortality of all living organisms. History demonstrates that we as a human race are no exception to our own mortal existence on this planet. The real miracle is the perpetuation of life, a conceived lineage of the past, currently you, and future generations. Your mortal framework is a mere vessel composed of universal forces, harnessed by your innate intelligence for the duration of your life. Innate forces are always constructive, preserving and protecting to sustain and maintain life. Adapting to, while manipulating universal forces, innate intelligence offers a more adequate model for articulating and understanding the potentially resilient and adaptive systems. Even in the face of destructive challenges, your innate forces overcome immeasurable odds for survival. By adopting the understanding that the world does not always work in a predictable manner, your internalized innate intelligence wages a war, a balancing act to preserve and perpetuate life. The small acorn, barring any interference, will become a majestic tree and produce more acorns to one day replace it, completing a universal cycle of life. The goal of a chiropractor is to ensure a balance of forces exist within you by removing any interference, allowing the innate to govern the universal components that comprise you. Chiropractors focus on the life-giving and constructive potential achieved when the innate has 100 percent communication to and from all parts of your body. Just as the acorn contains the mighty oak, you have everything that you need to live to your fullest potential while under regular chiropractic care.

Principle 26 reminds me that life on this earth is limited and that my innate intelligence is working this very minute in time to keep me alive, juggling the many life processes! This very minute, my innate is constructively safeguarding my life, maintaining homeostasis! Destructive universal forces are being beaten up and rejected as my internal innate forces succeed in giving to me the fullest expression of *life*! In closing, remember, small acorns grow and become mighty oak trees with the right nurturing.

Transformation
Dr. Daniel R. Constable, DC, ACP

• • •

Nothing is bigger than life.

—Dr. Sid E. Williams

Family—where life begins and love never ends.

—Author Unknown

Since I graduated from Palmer College of Chiropractic, the fountainhead of chiropractic, most people would imagine that I received the best chiropractic education money could buy. However, at the time of my graduation in October 2000, Palmer, like most chiropractic colleges and indeed the profession itself, was going through much turmoil, and both were firmly at the mercy of the Council on Chiropractic Education (CCE). As a result, my chiropractic education was in the end more of a "medipractic" education. I was taught how to adjust the spinal column, of course, but I was also drilled in physical therapy and rehabilitation. I was taught how to interpret blood and urine analyses, and there was a heavy emphasis on physical examination and diagnosis.

As a new graduate, I began my career as an independent contractor in a multi-doctor practice that was very much musculoskeletal pain syndrome oriented. The first eight years of my career, I spent diagnosing and treating headaches, neck aches, and low-back pain with a combination of adjusting, exercises, rehabilitation methods, nutritional support, and at times even psychological advice.

By the time I was in my early thirties, I had become quite successful in this diagnostic, therapeutic, mechanistic model of musculoskeletal pain syndrome treatment. However, I was not happy. I was tired. I was bored. I was burned out. I was faced with the question, "Is that it?" Is this what chiropractic is all about? In fact, I came closer than most people in my life to realize to quitting the profession because of a lack of motivation and desire to spend the rest of my life doing what I was doing.

As fate would have it, around this time, my father, Robert, was diagnosed with stage-four colon cancer. During a routine checkup with his medical doctor, a small amount of occult blood was found in his stool. A further array of tests revealed an orange-sized tumor in his distal colon. Overnight, my asymptomatic father was suddenly deathly ill.

When I found out Dad was sick, I went right into medi-practic mode, my modus operandi. I sent him books and cd´s about cancer and the recovery therefrom. I sent him supplements in pill and powder form. I called him regularly on the telephone and tried to help him or coach him as best I could. I was willing to do anything I possibly could to get dad well.

After a brave three-year battle, it was clear dad was going to lose his fight. I was lucky enough to spend the last three days of his life with him in a hospice in Melbourne, Australia, where I grew up. On the third day, the two of us finally had some time alone together, and at one stage, out of the blue, dad asked me, "Danny, do you think you could adjust me?" That moment remains the most ashamed I have ever been of myself in my entire life. Having been there three days and three nights, I had not even thought to offer to adjust him. So, I answered, "yes, of course."

Dad was bedridden by that stage and very stiff and immoveable, so I was very limited as to what I could do with him. However, I was able to palpate and analyze his neck. I discovered an upper cervical subluxation and adjusted him with the greatest of care. It remains the greatest adjustment I have ever given. I returned to the side of dad's bed and took his hand. After a minute of silence, he turned his head toward me, looked me directly in the eyes, and said, "Thank you." He then turned his head back to the middle, shut his eyes, and took a deep, cleansing breath, and he died.

A couple of days later, I was at my father's house, the house where I grew up, preparing for his funeral. I was looking through his wardrobe when I discovered at the back of the wardrobe on the floor all of the books, the cd's, and the pills and powders, everything I had been sending the previous three years, all still there and all still wrapped in the plastic wrapping I sent them in. Dad never read a book, never listened to a cd, and never took a pill or a powder. Dad's partner, Anne, was with me at the time, and she saw I was struggling to deal with what I was looking at. She came over to me, put a hand on my shoulder, and said, "You know, all he ever wanted was an adjustment." At the most difficult time of his life and at the moment of his death, dad was not interested in all of that other stuff. All of the other stuff I was doing for him and all of the other stuff I was doing for my patients in my practice, he was not interested in. All he ever wanted was an adjustment.

Dad's death and the days following were what taught me what chiropractic is really all about. Having had the privilege of being there in that moment when a human being passes on from this life to the next, I am convinced that we all have an innate desire to be in a state of connection when we leave this world—connection to ourselves, connection to our families, connection to our maker. There is something magical about the chiropractic adjustment. Chiropractic is not about pain. Dad didn't have any pain. Chiropractic is about connecting the brain to the body and the body to the brain. Chiropractic is about ensuring the nerve channels of the axial skeleton (the cranium, the spine, and the pelvis) remain open to allow for the better function of the nervous system. The practice of chiropractic is about the detection, analysis, and correction of vertebral subluxation for the better and optimal expression of life.

This, together with the conviction that everybody is better off without vertebral subluxation than with it, has transformed my practice and shaped the way I and my family lead our lives. I believe that as long as you have a brain and a spine, you belong in the hands of a chiropractor. Vertebral subluxation alone is reason enough to be regularly examined and if necessary adjusted by a chiropractor. There is no time when a human being is better off if left subluxated. As a result, it is imperative that every man, woman, and child incorporate chiropractic into their lives. The developer of chiropractic, Dr. B. J. Palmer, wrote of a chiropractic utopia. I believe the job of the chiropractor is to take care of his or her community, to leave his or her community less subluxated and therefore healthier and happier than how he or she found it. Imagine communities full of people more in tune with themselves, their families, their fellow humans, and their environment. Following my transformation from medipractor to chiropractor, this has become my purpose. Thank you, dad, for showing me with your death what my life is all about. Thank you for giving me my purpose. I miss you. I love you.

Simplicity is the key to brilliance.

—BRUCE LEE

PRINCIPLE 27

The Normality of Innate Intelligence
Andreas Soderstrom, DC, ACP, Sweden

● ● ●

Innate intelligence is always normal, and its function is always normal.

I BELIEVE THIS IS A central idea that separates us humans in a modern society, where either we think that for most part, we come into this world through an amazing journey governed by the body's inborn wisdom and we are perfect creatures just about to express ourselves over a lifetime through adaptation and by trusting the body's ability to cope with the forces and challenges thrown at us from simply being alive, or we believe that we are created with a need of help in order to survive and for the body to navigate itself in life through the means of outside interventions.

Principle 27 stems from the major premise of chiropractic, which acknowledges and identifies a universal power and intelligence, and these ideas lead me to believe that chiropractic is coming of age, for they seem to reflect the insights of our chiropractic forebears, especially those of B. J. Palmer, who was writing in the first part of the last century. In 1948, R. W. Stephenson set out B. J.'s thirty-three principles, and despite the fact that some practitioners today question the validity of these principles, they seem to resonate with many other disciplines today. The principles are holding the tests and could be guiding people in other areas than chiropractic.

One of the best chefs in the world, Dan Barber, known for Blue Hill at Stone Bars and Blue Hill New York, started what is referred to as the "farm-to-table movement" with his philosophy of creating great food. Dan Barber has understood that no matter how good your technique is in cooking food, if you don't have great ingredients, you cannot make great food. How does this relate to principle 27?

Dan Barber is on a mission to chase great flavors. When doing so, you chase the best ingredients, and then you are in search of great farming. He states, "As you go deeper into the symbiotic relationships in the biology of farming, you improve the grass, and if you improve the grass, you are improving every bite the dairy cows are eating, and if you are improving that, you are improving the milk." He knows that to support the continuation of the whole system is the goal for better flavor. What is a carrot that is the essence of a carrot?

You cannot taste great flavor unless the soil is a fully active biological community. All we know for sure is that the more life we have in the soil, the more potential we have for the creation of great taste. He also says that you are what you eat, but you are what *what you eat* eats too. This is an opportunity to teach people to be thinking not only on what they eat but also what *what they eat* is eating. This to me is another idea on what a chef or restaurant can be because it aims to teach people about a message bigger than the actual food on the plate. A gift from nature could be that when you treat nature well; it gives you the gift of great food.

With this in mind, let's look at the major premise, which states that a universal intelligence is in all matter and continually gives to it all its properties and actions, thus maintaining it in existence. This is the first principle that all the other principles are deduced from. May it then be that the search for great flavors is simply the search for each ingredient's normal being, created with no interference from outside sources but instead governed by its innate intelligence, which results in what resonates with us humans as great taste and even an extraordinary plate of food.

Could we use this principle as the canvas to broadcast ideas that will influence people in a way that goes hand in hand with the chiropractic principles? I believe it already does.

For a chiropractic practice, I think it is vital to have full trust in principle 27 because it sets the tone for the entire expression of chiropractic.

33

Clarence Gonstead used to say, "Never question the principle of chiropractic but question the application of chiropractic." When you understand innate intelligence is always normal and always at 100 percent, you also understand it does what it is supposed to with the forces it has to deal with. When you remove any interference to innate intelligence, it can express itself normally. The mind-set a chiropractor adopts knowing this is to focus on the objective (subluxation) and not the outcome. Therefore, you also become, as a practitioner, more present and specific when adjusting a subluxation because you honor the organized intelligence and you are doing your best to guide the innate in what is supposed to be done when adjusting a subluxation. Going back to the chef looking to find the best taste, we can see he understands the power of nature creating this by letting the ingredients be as natural (normal) as possible, and with this, he can develop the craft of cooking. Only with the understanding that innate is always normal can we develop the craft of adjusting as chiropractors.

It is not our job as chiropractors to judge the normal expression of innate intelligence; rather, we should pay attention to that.

To lay-people, I explain this principle in many different ways, and most often, I do that when people are worried about different symptoms that are just physiological responses or adaptations run by innate intelligence and in fact a sign of being healthy and not sick. When children have fever, it is a normal response, trying to bring the entire system into homeostasis by raising body temperature to take care of foreign viruses or bacteria that may not survive in the heated environment. It is therefore vital for us as chiropractors to inform people we meet about the basis of our principles. Most parents would give their children medications to lower the fever and by doing so are interfering with a normal and natural process that needs to take place. To me, this is a great opportunity to educate people about a different paradigm in today's society, and when explaining it from this perspective, people's perception of health may change, and they may become more careful of judging what takes place in a healthy response called sickness.

Another example I use in practice is that your blood calcium levels must always remain within a normal range, determined by your body's intelligence. Should your levels drop too low, your parathyroid glands know how to obtain calcium from your bones and deposit it into your blood. When it comes to blood pressure, people are taught to believe it always has to stay in a certain range, and if it does not, most likely, they take prescribed drugs, not looking for the reasons behind too high or low pressure. In fact, it is just a normal response adapting to the challenges put forth by the environment, like stress or obesity. People will still die from heart failure being on blood-pressure medications. The laws governed by innate intelligence determine how things in your body should happen and what we need to listen and pay attention to.

In my personal life, principle 27 brings me closer to nature and things natural, and in a modern world, I sometimes feel like the chef chasing the greatest flavor by moving toward nature as much as possible. By removing manmade toxins that interfere with my very being and by investing time in nature, I feel connected with my normal expression of innate intelligence. In my practice, I want people to leave after the adjustment feeling more connected with the normal (nature).

33

This next principle has very special meaning because of the circumstances surrounding its author and submission. Dr. Andy Roberts was a fellow Delta Sigma Chi brother and was an online friend. We never officially met in person, but I have and had great respect for this man's vision and dedication to a principle greater than himself.

Andy had sent me his submission one day before his passing. We had spoken on the phone that morning and he was in great spirits and excited to come to do a seminar we had been planning with him in Argentina.

His life was one of legacy, and he will be forever remembered for his teachings, dedication, and inspiration of others to master their craft. Thank you, Andy, for the life you lived and what you stood for.

PRINCIPLE 28

The Conductors of Innate Forces
Andy Roberts, DC

• • •

The forces of innate intelligence operate through or over the nervous system in animal bodies.

THE HUMAN BEING IS A marvelous and mysterious design in structure and function. Despite all the years of study, billions of dollars spent, brilliant minds thinking, and the development of cutting-edge technologies that have been used to study the human being, we still know only an inkling of our capabilities. While the brain, heart, liver, eyes, spleen, and the other individual parts and organs are each wonders of function, we are so much more than the sum of those parts. We comprise a collection of machine parts working together for the greater good of the entire being, all coordinated through the nervous system by the body's inborn wisdom, which chiropractors call innate intelligence.

Not too far from where I live is the University of Michigan (U of M), home to one of the largest sports stadiums in the world. Imagine for a moment, the U of M stadium is filled to capacity with over 107,000 people filling the seats. You are there, standing smack dab in the middle of the field, and you are asked to perform but one task. That one task is to convey to each of the 107,000 people a simple piece of information, an instruction to do something and then receive back from each a message on the performance of that task. How long would you need? How long would it take to accomplish this task—days, weeks, or perhaps even months or longer? As simple as the instruction might be, this seems to be a daunting if not

33

an impossible feat to achieve. But now imagine if I told you that you didn't have all that time, that you only had a moment in time, perhaps even less than a second to communicate your message to all of the 107,000! Forget about it! Shut down the system, turn off the stadium lights, and let's go home. I have a difficult enough time coordinating my four children!

Would you be amazed that this complex-type communication happens within you from the moment of your conception to your very last breath, but on an even grander and more incredible scale? Your body is made up of approximately thirty-seven trillion cells. Each of these thirty-seven trillion cells requires a unique message every moment for it to carry out its function and sustain your life. A skin cell on your pinky toe and a cell in your heart and all the other cells in between need to carry out their unique functions while contributing to that of the whole body. Fortunately, we don't have to do the football-stadium-type exercise, and, thankfully, we don't need to think about the control and coordination of our thirty-seven trillion cells either. We have innate intelligence to do it for us.

While we busy ourselves with school, work, and play; while we worry about the weather, finances, and global peace; while we sleep, wake, eat, and drink, innate intelligence is diligently and relentlessly on the job, receiving the needs and demands of the body and formulating the appropriate action, relaying the discrete and unique message to each and every cell and then once again receiving feedback to begin the cycle again. This is accomplished moment to moment, over and over again for your entire life. Without even the slightest attention or thought in your mind, a stomach-lining cell, a hormone-producing gland cell, and a colon-wall cell are receiving and sending messages in order to successfully carry out their functions and coordinated action for the good of the whole.

In the sport's stadium, it would have been quite futile for you to stand on the field and shout your commands. Even the closest of people would have a hard time hearing you, let alone those in the nosebleed seats. It makes sense that you would need a communication system, perhaps a microphone, that you could speak into, which would direct your commands sent over 107,000 wires designated for each and every person in the language he or she understands. Your body is no different. The innate intelligence that controls, regulates, and coordinates each and every one of your thirty-seven trillion cells needs a way by which it can communicate its messages. This is your nervous system.

Let's take a moment to appreciate the wonder of your nervous system. It was the first structure to form from a ball of undifferentiated cells soon after fertilization of the egg. Nerve cells called neurons grow at the rate of 250,000 neurons a minute while still in the womb. The sheer size and network of this system is such that if you stripped away everything of the body except for the nervous system, you would undeniably see the structure of the human form. Some nerve cells can conduct a signal at a rate of more than three hundred feet per second!

The messages of innate intelligence are called mental impulses and innate forces. They are transmitted from your brain over the conductors (nerves) of your body to the receivers (tissue cells) to cause a desired function. Once the cell has received the message, a status report is sent back via conductors (nerves) to the brain where the cycle starts all over again. If this cycle from brain cell to tissue cell is occurring unimpeded, as it should in all the cycles for each cell of the body, then we are expressing our maximum potential of health and life.

If, however, there is an impedance of the messages, which are vital for the cell to carry out its functions, an altered state of being occurs, which we refer to as disease. When disease occurs, the cell, tissue, organ, system, and ultimately the body enters a state of disharmony, rendering it unable to function adequately and unable to adapt properly to its environment. If left in this condition, over time (and sometimes immediately), a myriad of problems may occur (some we name and classify as one disease or another). Chiropractic names the impedance (block of flow of mental impulse) within the nerve cycles due to misaligned vertebrae a *vertebral subluxation*.

When a bone of the spine misaligns because of any one or combination of reasons, it can alter the neurology of the body and negatively affect the flow of the mental impulses and innate forces. This is the vertebral subluxation. As you can imagine, vertebral subluxation is always bad, and you would always want to be free of it. Let's use an example most all of us can relate to on some level.

Think for a moment about the various systems of your car—the cooling system, the drivetrain, the electrical system, the brake lines, and more. We will skip the obvious example of the electrical system and use the brake lines to truly bring home the seriousness of this problem. In most conventional cars with disk brakes, fluid is circulated from the master cylinder into the brake assembly at the wheels, which makes the two brake pads squeeze together against the rotor, causing the wheels to slow and eventually stop. Here's the scary part: imagine that while you are driving, the brake line that carries the fluid gets compromised in a way that diminishes the fluid flow or, worse, cut completely, resulting in total loss of all the fluid in the brake line! Now as you are pleasantly driving along, approaching a red light, unexpected traffic, or a sharp turn, you put your foot down on the brake pedal and you get the surprise of your life—no brakes! No need to go into the details of the horrors of the outcome. I'm sure you all understand what can happen.

The vertebral subluxation is to your body what the compromised line is to the braking system of your car. Remember, every single part of your body has a supply line—your heart, liver, lungs, reproductive organs, and every other organ as well! If any of these supply lines have a "compromise" in them, you can imagine the devastation in terms of function, performance, and life that would cause to the organs they supply.

Chiropractic principle 28 states that the forces of innate intelligence operate through or over the nervous system in animal bodies. Without the conductors of innate forces working properly, we cease to function normally, and we may, ultimately, die.

Crush your Comfort Zone

• • •

*The best things in life are often waiting for you
at the exit ramp of your comfort zone.*

—Karen Salmanshon

*If you put yourself in a position where you have
to stretch yourself out of your comfort zone, then
you are forced to expand your consciousness.*

—Les Brown

Anyone who has ever made massive impact will tell you that most of the time they spend breaking comfort zones, entering into new ones, and repeating the cycle. My family lives in Palm Beach Gardens, Florida, about ten minutes from some of the most beautiful beaches in the world. Yet I knew for me to grow, I had to step into the unknown, which is part of what drove me to leave this comfortable paradise and go to South America, specifically Argentina, during the country's worst crisis in history. My path since taking that step has been one of major discomfort yet exponential growth in every human way possible.

According to major studies on human life, 90 percent of humans get to the end of their lives with major regrets. Very often, that is because they stayed within their comfort zone on so many levels. They stayed in the same town they were born

33

in, stayed in relationships or jobs that didn't work, and so on. The list is endless. No matter what age you are, where you live, your economic status, or how you currently practice, it is never too late to step out of the comfortable box you have created and make more impact.

We are brainwashed to believe life should be comfortable and easy. Most successful people will tell you that it is the hard times that build character. Once you start breaking down your barriers of comfort you will find this is where where the true evolution of "you" takes place.

> **The comfort zone is the great enemy to creativity; moving beyond it necessitates intuition, which in turn configures new perspectives and conquers fears.**
>
> —Dan Stevens

PRINCIPLE 29

Interference with the Transmission of Innate Forces
Dan Sullivan, DC

● ● ●

There can be interference with the transmission of innate forces.

FIRST AND FOREMOST, THE PREVIOUS two principles describe the quality and importance of biological forces. Internal biological forces are always striving for adaptation. In other words, the body is smarter than our educated mind and therefore always doing the right thing at the right time. Symptoms, although unwanted in most circumstances, are an expression of the body adapting to the environmental forces in a perfect way. Second, we know that environmental forces are destructive, but internal innate biological forces are constructive to the specific living thing that creates them. Innate intelligence creates the forces in a living body that are always adapting with a constructive force intended for survival of that organism—unless the internal biological forces suffer interference.

The public can understand the concept of interference if explained appropriately. Three examples represent and clearly drive home how the transmission of internal biological processes can have interference: plaque buildup in an artery, a fractured bone, and a tumor. An artery with plaque buildup can interfere with the flow of blood so much that it can create death. A bone can withstand significant pressure and force, but a limit exists. When the limit of a bone is overcome, a fracture can occur. And many times, a fractured bone must be set back into a proper healing position to regain as much normal motion and function as possible. Or a tumor in any part of the body can compress vital areas that interfere with

33

life-giving processes. For instance, a tumor on a nerve or blood vessel, on the spinal cord, or in a lung creates interference to the normal expression of biological processes.

Notice that these are examples of interference with normal biological processes but are applicable to the principle that innate forces can be interfered with. However, there is a difference between biological processes and biological forces. Our founders and early pioneers defined processes different from forces to uniquely distinguish the qualities of the mental impulse from a simple body function or nerve-action potential. This is important in order for us to understand the implications of a subluxation that interferes with the mental impulse and the profound influence of an adjustment to restore function by removing interference from the mental impulse.

Without the understanding and explanation that this principle lays out, the need for chiropractic and the adjustment would be of little value. The fact that interference can occur with the transmission of internal biological forces explains why the necessity for correction of vertebral subluxation remains so vital to the expression of human life and potential in the world today. Interference with the internal biological forces occurs because of the limitations of the matter, not because of the limitation of intelligence. Without the possibility for interference with the biological forces through the constraints of matter, the subluxation or need for the chiropractic adjustment does not exist.

This principle lays the groundwork for why a subluxation poses a unique threat to the expression of life and the human experience. As described in previous principles, innate intelligence is always at 100 percent. Therefore, the quality of innate forces cannot be interfered with. But the quantity of internal biological forces can be interfered with because of their relationship with matter. All internal innate biological forces must be expressed in matter. And all matter is susceptible to its constraints. From principle 5, we know that all humans need 100 percent of intelligence, force, and matter to flawlessly exist. Described by principle 24, we know that matter is the weakest of the triune (intelligence, force, matter). As structure and function are intimately connected, any structural weakness will have a significant effect on its ability to function. Tissue cells (matter) will fail if the stresses for adaptation move beyond their physical limitations. Like a broken bone or tumor, this is the significance of interference. If the interference cannot be corrected or removed, function and survival of the organism are reduced.

A fever, high blood pressure, and diarrhea are examples of how the body is always doing the right thing at the right time. Symptoms are a perfect expression of biological processes adapting to the environment. Innate intelligence constantly seeks to adapt, heal, and repair. But when inference occurs with normal innate biological forces, the ability for the body to adapt, regulate, and repair is altered. Interference with innate forces leads to dysfunction and disease. Over time, unwanted symptoms are the result of undetected and uncorrected interferences in the body.

Correction of the interference is necessary for the expression of force through matter to be normal again. The disappearance of symptoms because of the correction of subluxation, as seen in chiropractors' offices around the world each week, is a perfect example of how this principle applies to life. Interference is real and possible. And although the intelligence in matter is perfect, the matter itself has constraints and limitations. When interference occurs, life is not expressed at its full potential. Chiropractors help every man, woman, and child experience their full potential by removing interference with the transmission of internal biological forces with the adjustment.

Craft

• • •

> You can never let anything distract you from your main objective. My only goal is to be great. That's all I want. That's all I aspire to be. Greatness is something nobody can ever take away from you, no matter what happens. So I put all of my energy and focus into my craft.
>
> —Larry Fitzgerald

> If flipping hamburgers at McDonald's, be the best hamburger flipper in the world. Whatever it is you do, you have to master your craft.
>
> —Snoop Dogg

A CRAFT IS AN ACTIVITY *involving skill in making things by hand. Chiropractors are philosophers, scientists, artists, marketers, businesspeople, and teachers to name of a few of the skill sets we need to have in order to thrive. I like to think of it all as a craft. We are using our hands to work, and although we don't make objects, we enhance life expression through removing vertebral subluxations. That is craftsmenship at its finest.*

Science shows that it takes ten thousand hours to become a master. That is in the context that we are doing everything in a skilled, diligent way; otherwise, we become masters at mediocrity. I think back to when B. J. Palmer and Gonstead were alive. They spent countless hours perfecting their craft. Their craft consumed every ounce of their being and world.

The responsibility we have as Doctors of Chiropractic is tremendous. We are dealing with people's lives. We adjust the physiological and physical center of the human being, the spine. We must be vigilant in our responsibility to accurately analyze the spine in a sacred and humanistic yet scientific way. I remember Thom Gelardi telling me that learning our craft is a lifetime venture. I have had the fortune to meet and be mentored by masters in chiropractic, and the seriousness, professionalism, and dedication they put into mastering every aspect of our craft is astounding.

It has been said by great scientists and philosophers that the greater our sphere of understanding becomes, the greater the sphere of the unknown becomes, and on and on. So learning and mastery become a constant evolution of gaining knowledge, experience, and wisdom and then not knowing once again until we evolve to knowing on a deeper level and gain more profound wisdom, knowledge, and experience until this cycle repeats itself over and over for our lifetime.

The only true wisdom is knowing you know nothing.

—SOCRATES

PRINCIPLE 30

The Causes of Dis-ease
Kari Swain, DC

• • •

Interference with the transmission of innate forces causes incoordination of dis-ease.

FROM PRINCIPLE 12, WE KNOW that there can be interference with the transmission of universal forces. There are many examples in the world, such as a wall blocking the wind and a lead apron blocking x-rays.

Soon after the discovery of chiropractic, D. D. Palmer and B. J. Palmer, along with his inner circle of chiropractors, including Craven, Vedder, Firth, Burich, and Mabel Palmer, were busy developing its philosophy. They used common words of the day but with their own spin on their definitions as well as new words they created to aid in the explanation of the concepts and constructs of chiropractic. To set the stage, it is important to realize the distinct definitions of the lexicon used.

Dis-ease is the cause of much confusion to both the chiropractor and the layperson, as it is often thought to be synonymous with *disease*, which couldn't be further from the truth. Before we talk about *dis-ease* and the difference with *disease*, the concept of *ease* as used in chiropractic must be clear. In the modern dictionary, the word is simply defined as freedom from labor, pain, or physical annoyance; tranquil rest; or comfort. R. W. Stephenson said, "In chiropractic, ease is the entity…" The entity that is "ease" is the completeness of a person, and it can be seen in the various words used to describe it, such as *health*, *adaptation*, *coordination*, and well-being. On the simplest level, the communication between a single brain cell and tissue cell, the use of *ease*, in the vernacular, is normal function of the body and each tissue cell and each cell carrying out its duty.

Dis-ease, then, in its most simplistic form, is the lack of ease. It is a deviation from the maintenance of the balanced functioning of all the interrelated parts of the body. This deviation is the result of the disruption of communication between the brain and the body.

The converse of *ease* is *dis-ease*. In chiropractic, we put a hyphen into the word itself to stand for less than ease. In essence, a word may seem to be common but has a different meaning in the chiropractic realm. The *Merriam-Webster Dictionary* defines *disease* as "an illness that affects a person, animal or plant, a condition that prevents the body or mind from working normally; a problem that a person, group, organization, or society cannot stop."

Chiropractic dis-ease is the incoordination of the innate forces. Those innate forces are constructive, not destructive. Innate forces are responsible for the function and repair of the tissue.

According to Stephenson's text, *incoordination* is the lack of harmony in the actions of the body, due to the lack of innate control. It is the condition of unbalanced service or rather the unbalanced actions of tissue cells, which then fail. The actions of the tissue cells are not coordinative service unless they act in obedience to the law of demand and supply (principle 33). Incoordination is called dis-ease because tissue cells will become unsound when they are neglected by the organization.

In the dictionary explanation, *incoordination* is the more global sense of the inability to use the different parts of the body together smoothly and efficiently. Palmer and his fellows really were indicating the incoordination with the brain to the tissue cell. Incoordination is when the cycle between brain and tissue cell or the message is not getting through or is altered or changed and that puts us in the state of dis-ease.

Coordination is when every demand from the brain to the tissue is getting through; if we have coordination, we have a state of ease.

The normal state of being is supposed to be ease. By design, we are born to be healthy. It is our birthright to have innate intelligence on the job to manifest the fullest expression of life. Living in the physical world, one is exposed to physical forces; these are universal forces. Universal forces are always destructive. Matter is continuously adapting to those outside forces. The healthier the matter, the easier it is for the matter to adapt to those forces. An example of a universal force is gravity. Regardless of where you are, gravity is always working.

The body has all the potential that is necessary for the successful transmission of the innate forces unless there is interference. There are many things that can cause interference of the transmission of those innate forces. The cause chiropractors are most concerned with is the vertebral subluxation. When present, the vertebral subluxation interferes with the transmission of the mental impulses. That interference affects the body's ability to heal itself.

Any interference with the transmission of innate intelligence will cause a change in cell coordination and motion. This, in turn, alters adaptation and results in what chiropractors call dis-ease. Any change of vibration in the transmission of the mental impulse will cause the tissue cells to receive an altered mental impulse. These cells will then act out of coordination, allowing the destructive universal forces to act on the tissue cells and result in dysfunction, disharmony, and dis-ease. Any alteration in the flow of mental force will result in an alteration in the adaptability of a complex structure or organism.

The universal forces of autosuggestions (thoughts), toxins, and traumas all combine to negatively impact the function of the nervous system. Restoration of ease is only gained from within the body by removing the interference in the transmission. Specific chiropractic analysis and adjustment to the vertebral subluxation removes the interference and restores the transmission of innate intelligence.

The design of the body is brilliant. The system has backup plans built into the "operating system." Those built-in redundancies allow for adaptation to universal forces throughout life. However, those backup plan systems were never meant for sustaining the human being indefinitely.

The US interstate system is also an amazing design. In 1956, President Eisenhower signed the federal-aid highway act. The interstate system now has 46,876 miles of roadway. In total, the United States has over four million miles of roads. That is a lot of streets and highways!

Consider two major interstates just down the road from where I practice. Interstate 80 spans the width of the entire United States and intersects with Interstate 35. That runs from Canada to the southernmost point in Texas. Many times, a construction zone or accident of some sort will cause traffic to be rerouted until the repair is done and the road is cleared. Sometimes even weather can cause detours or a section of the road to be shut down. The road is still there, though the travel on the roads is limited to emergency vehicles and snowplows. For normal travelers, an alternate route will work. Sometimes, an alternate route is not available, perhaps because a blizzard has shut all routes down around the interstates as well. Now, a traveler with any sense isn't going to hunker down in the car for the night, as he or she might freeze to death. He or she will find a roadside motel or alternate lodging until the storm passes. However, a traveler who believes he or she knows better than the controlling system will disobey the rules and try to push through, often creating a disaster. Now connect how the body has episodes of rerouting or recruiting alternative pathways until adaptation or restoration can occur. Those processes can be limited when the traveler decides to try to override the Department of Transportation, the governing system, not allowing the backup plans to work (taking alternative routes or holding up for the duration of the storm). A specific chiropractic adjustment is like sending a snowplow to the location of snow drifted over traffic lanes. It clears the path for the traveler. On the same note, if that snowplow runs down the road with its blade engaged, it could scrape up and cause damage to the roadway, again causing a detour for the traveler. Apply that concept to a non-specific adjustment, sending destructive universal forces into the nervous system.

Unfortunately, sometimes the Department of Transportation knows there is a problem and underestimates its severity or overlooks it, as was the case in the collapse of the Interstate 35 bridge in Minneapolis in 2007. Small patchwork repairs had been made, but the structural integrity was damaged and that had catastrophic effects for the travelers on and around the road. By not addressing the bombardment of universal forces and way more traffic than the system was designed for and not having adequate alternate routes (internal backup systems in the body), the Department of Transportation had a catastrophe on their hands. The same holds true for the traveler who fails to adapt; dis-ease is the effect.

The brilliance of the interstate system was scoffed at in its inception in 1956. Now, it is widely accepted as one of the greatest conveniences in road travel. Think about going anywhere in your car across the country without an interstate!

The cause of dis-ease as it relates to the detection and correction of the vertebral subluxation and the way that the interference from the subluxation causes a change in the adaptability of the matter. In the specific adjustment, the interference is removed and the body function restored. The full expression of innate intelligence is possible when there is no vertebral subluxation present, creating interference between the brain and the tissue cell, leading to the incoordination of dis-ease. The specific adjustment of the vertebral subluxation is the one and only job of a chiropractor.

Choices

● ● ●

Intelligence is the ability to adapt to change.

—Stephen Hawking

Natural ability is important but you can go far without it, if you have the focus, drive, desire and positive attitude.

—Kirsten Sweetland

At every second, at every turn, you have choices. You are in your power and create life, or you complain and destroy life. You live at a high vibration, winning, learning, growing, and evolving, or you lose. You create new possibilities, or you waste precious time. You have gratitude for everyone and everything or become a victim of circumstance. As Tony Robbins says, attraction comes when we are living a high vibration and are grateful and positive. If we have expectations, then we expect them to be met, and when they are not, we become resentful, complain, and lose our ability to attract.

33

Create your life, or complain your life. The choice is yours. Any and every situation or circumstance you are living can either create possibility or destroy it. Winners either win, or they learn, grow, adapt, and evolve.

**Success is on the same road as failure; success
is just a little further down the road.**

—JACK HYLES

PRINCIPLE 31

Subluxations
Rob Sinnot, DC, DPhCS

• • •

Interference with transmission in the body is always directly or indirectly due to subluxations in the spinal column.

As do all principles designed in a formal logic model, this principle is dependent upon and deduced from the preceding principles. Thus far, we have explored the character of innate forces, the transmission of innate forces, and the understanding that there can be interference with those innate forces. The innate forces in this respect are the mental impulses. These are perfect, without exception. We know this, as innate intelligence is always perfect, and its function—the creation of mental impulses from assembled foruns in this case—can be no exception. This means that when there is an interference with the flow of mental impulse supply from the brain to the tissue cell, it is *always* one of *quantity* and can *never* be one of *quality*. If it were possible to interfere with the quality, it would no longer be perfect and by definition would not be a mental impulse but a common universal force.

As we consider the concept of interference with the quantity of the flow of mental-impulse supply, we must recognize the type of interference as it relates to the vertebral subluxation. The vertebral subluxation has qualifying characteristics that have been abbreviated often in discussion, but it is vital to comprehend them as they were philosophically intended. Too often, we see the inclination to blur the lines of our philosophy in order to allow a larger tent to include things not intended to be chiropractic within our philosophy. This action does no justice to the purity of our chiropractic philosophy and spreads confusion through the profession. The first rule in frank discussion is to define our terms. Fortunately, *vertebral subluxation* was defined long before any of us set foot in the profession. The four components described by B. J. Palmer and laid out in Stephenson's 1927 tome are even more scientifically supportable today than they were in that era.

First, we recognize the vertebral subluxation is defined by a loss of juxtaposition with the vertebra above, below, or both. The second component is the accompanying occlusion of a neural foramen that necessarily occurs with the loss of proper alignment. Third, the change in form of the neural foramen in question will result in a change in function for the transmitting foramen. When you alter the form of anything from its original manner, you by definition will alter its function as well. As we know, function follows form. This may result in our third component: compromised neural integrity or function. In D. D. Palmer's words, "Structure and function, normal or abnormal, go together. Function is dependent upon structure."

At this point, we have briefly touched upon the first three components. We do not have a vertebral subluxation but a simple neuropathy. It is the fourth—the interference with the quantity of the flow of mental impulses—that needs the most detailed explanation.

When the term *mental impulse* was coined, it was used for a specific and very important reason. At the time, the nerve impulse was being discussed in neurology and physiology. It was thought at that time that the nerve impulse fell short of what was being observed. Think of it this way. Even today, we know that there are various forms of neural communication accepted under the definition of the nerve impulse. There are membrane polarization-depolarization, vesicle transport, and other standard views being taught in our schools, as they are in medical schools. Together, they cannot account for the speed our brains function at. The field of science is working diligently, and one day, they may have defined this to mathematical satisfaction. As for today, they have not yet arrived.

Our founders felt that the use of the term *mental impulse* and the description of it as *abstract* were necessary. If they were to use the *nerve impulse* as it was understood in 1927, for example, they knew science would find that to be a poor definition at some point in the near future. They reasoned that if they were to adhere to the nerve impulse and science discarded that theory when new data arrived to better explain the phenomenon, they could be seen as adhering to worthless antiquated science. For this reason, they coined the term *mental impulse* and had to make it abstract, as science had not yet determined what they knew must be true. They stated that at such a time when science can properly define the communicative ability they knew to be present, they could discard *mental impulse* and use the new term of that time. That time has yet to come.

Sadly, our profession knows little of this historical rationale that still holds just as accurate today. An important feature of the mental impulse is its role. The mental impulse provides instructions for adaptation for a given moment in time and a given set of circumstances.

This means the fourth component can be deduced by its function. There must be a loss of adaptability recognized in the tissue cell for a vertebral subluxation to be identified. When a patient presents with the first three components and an identifiable loss of adaptability, it can then be referred to as a vertebral subluxation. It is just as acceptable to measure the fourth component by its effects as it is to measure blood pressure with a cuff and stethoscope. These items do not measure blood pressure; they measure expansion at the skin surface assumed to be due to the heartbeat distal to it, causing the distension. This does not mean it is not a valid measurement, any more than that considered to determine the diminishment of the abstract mental-impulse flow. Both are rational and logical conclusions.

The vertebral subluxation initiates the downstream effects along the neuromere. The vertebral subluxation in this way introduces a special type of incoordination that can only be due to a vertebral subluxation named dis-ease. By definition, this incoordination may only result from a vertebral subluxation, as we see in viewing this principle in light of the one directly preceding it.

The vertebral subluxation is a cornerstone of our existence, and it must be grasped at an intimate level by those who desire to practice chiropractic.

33

Long and deliberate study is necessary to offer the best chiropractic service to your community. When I approach what I see as a problem of our philosophy, I first assume it is due to something I do not yet properly understand. It is that important step that we must all take when we undertake the path of our philosophy. Several decades later, I have yet to find that my initial view of a problem in our philosophy I encountered was not due to my own shortcomings. Most often, I find myself back at this list of thirty-three principles, using them as a compass to find my way to true north.

The Four Levels of Influence

• • •

If your actions inspire others to dream more, learn more, do more, and become more, you are a leader.

—John Quincy Adams

Amateurs spend most of their time designing slides to educate the room; professionals spend most of their time rehearsing their presentation to influence the room.

—Robert Monaco

I believe as chiropractors we have four basic levels of influence on people's decision making. Our energy can at times be aligned more with one level than another, while at other times, we can be a mixture of different levels. We may move up the levels, start directly in one level, or move back down the levels. The key is to understand the consciousness and specific results that each level will bring to our practices.

Level 1—Existence, Continued Survival (Wikipedia)
Everything in the practice and in the chiropractors life is in basic fight or flight, survival mode. There is no real energy behind the work. For example,

you walk into the practice, and the assistant acts as if there is no difference whether you are there or not. The brochures are old and outdated. The chiropractor does not take the time to educate the public about the principles of chiropractic. Everything is simply existing. These practices are in survival mode financially and have very little impact in making any real contribution to their community.

LEVEL 2—EDUCATOR-AN EDUCATOR IS A PERSON WHO HELPS OTHERS ACQUIRE KNOWLEDGE (WIKIPEDIA).
The "educator" takes the time to explain what chiropractic is and what it is not. At this level, the assistant takes on a bigger role than that of secretary. He or she becomes a part of the educational process. The focus of the educator is on the perfect power point presentation, brochure, system, and so on. The focus is on the presentation rather than the energy and delivery behind it. The educator is typically doing most of the talking rather than engaging people in the conversation. At level 2, we can develop a decent practice, but real influence and power only come when we reach the next level.

The level 1 and 2 practice members tend to choose chiropractic from their educated mind more than anything else. People can easily be persuaded away from their original decision simply by speaking with a friend, family member, or other professional. Levels 1 and 2 will not generate a great deal of referrals, and we find ourselves constantly looking for new people. Everything feels more forced, and we tend to have to repeat and enforce basic things, like following care plans, the purpose of chiropractic, why they should bring their children, and so on.

LEVEL 3—INSPIRER-AN INSPIRER FILLS ONE WITH AN ANIMATING, QUICKENING, OR EXALTING INFLUENCE (WIKIPEDIA).
When you get to level 3, you focus on the delivery of the information as well as the information itself. You realize how important the energy, tonality, and vibration of communication is in influencing people to make life-changing decisions. This level leads one to understand that as a chiropractor, you are only as good as your last visit. This level moves people who come to you from the inside out, and

they will be making their decisions on how you make them feel rather than their educated mind. When you inspire people, they tend to take more responsibility for being regular with care, bringing their children, referring others, and so on. You won't have to work as hard to generate an inside-out referral-based practice once you hit the level of "inspirer."

LEVEL 4—REVOLUTIONARY-REVOLUTIONARY MEANS INVOLVING OR CAUSING A COMPLETE OR DRAMATIC CHANGE (*WIKIPIDEA*).
Very few chiropractors on the planet ever become revolutionaries. Becoming a revolutionary takes a level of discipline, sacrifice, and commitment to a cause that very few are willing to take on. When you are in the presence of a revolutionary, your entire being shifts, and it's obvious that there is something profound about the person in your presence. By their very nature, revolutionaries are able to influence people at the deepest level. Typically, many people receiving chiropractic in a revolutionary's practice end up becoming chiropractors themselves.

> **I'm a great believer in luck, and I find the harder I work, the more I have of it.**
>
> —THOMAS JEFFERSON

PRINCIPLE 32

The Principle of Coordination
Liam Schubel, DC

● ● ●

Coordination is the principle of the harmonious action of all the parts of an organism in fulfilling their offices and purposes.

How would you explain this principle to a layperson?
IN CHIROPRACTIC, WE OPERATE FROM the premise that all parts in the body exist for a reason. Each body part plays a crucial role for all other body parts. When operating in unison and at 100 percent perfect function, our experience is one of optimal health and well-being.

While there are certain body parts that we can live without, all are necessary for optimal function. The more science advances, the more we learn just how important it is to keep all your body parts and of course keep them working optimally.

Years ago, in medical science, the thought was quite different. Body parts like the appendix, tonsils, and ovaries were thought to be optional organs and were routinely taken out in operations both to treat symptoms and as a means of preventing problems in the future.

Modern science, of course, has realized the importance of all these organs to optimal health. The appendix and tonsils have been found to be important to the optimal functioning of the immune system. The ovaries, of course, produce vital hormones for calcium absorption and cardiovascular health.

Body chemistry is crucial to the optimal functioning and well-being. Almost every process in the body is a chemical process. Digestion occurs in the stomach with the production of acids. The gallbladder produces bile for the chemical breakdown of fats. Brain chemistry largely determines our mood and energy levels. The pharmaceutical industry has spent trillions of dollars on the development of drugs that are used to manipulate the chemical processes of our bodies in an attempt to restore health.

Sadly, each of these synthetic chemicals has negative secondary effects. The body's intelligence can recognize the synthetic version and thus perceives the chemical as an attacker or a toxin. In addition, medical science has no way of knowing *exactly* how much chemical to introduce at *exactly* the right time. Too much chemical and we have created a less-than-optimal condition within the body. Too little chemical and we have also created a less-than-optimal condition as well.

What organ coordinates the seemingly magical interplay between *all* the organ systems of the body? The brain. How does it do it? Through a complex system of nerves.

Without this constant interplay between the brain and the other organs and systems, we simply begin to lose our ability to function optimally. If we disconnected the liver, the stomach, and the gallbladder from the central nervous system for example, how would the stomach know that it was full so the person would stop eating? How would the liver know what enzymes to produce and how much? How would the gallbladder know if a fatty meal had been eaten and thus there was a need for more bile?

As you can see, coordination is vital to the optimal human experience. It is our nerve system and the inborn intelligence within us that make all this coordination possible.

How does this principle apply to VS and practice?

Many times, practice members come to us with the desire to "treat" certain conditions. The unique role, however, of chiropractic is not to stimulate or inhibit body function through adjusting the spine. Instead, we liberate the nervous system so that the innate intelligence of the body may be expressed optimally. This in essence sets the body up for its greatest level of natural coordination.

Imagine trying to coordinate anything properly using an obstructed system of communication. Treating the effects of a body that has lost its optimal coordination is the role of medicine. Stimulating and inhibiting body-organ function and chemistry is the role of pharmaceutical prescriptions. Chiropractic's greatest achievement is restoring the body's optimal capacity to coordinate its functions. When this occurs, we can reach our greatest health and healing potential.

How does this principle apply to life?

In life, we find that the most successful systems are the ones that have the best communication and therefore the greatest level of effective coordination.

Can you give some examples of this principle in action?

Great examples of this are successful businesses and sports teams. You cannot have excellent coordination without excellent communication. The two go hand in hand.

When working to optimize a business, for example, the first thing most managers do is find out how people within the organization communicate and where that communication is breaking down. Once they have determined the blockages, they develop a strategy to remove them. The result is a more efficient and greater level of coordination. This leads to optimal results.

In the realm of team sports, coordination within the team is vital to winning. Each member plays a crucial role in the optimal performance of the team. You may have heard the adage "There is no *I* in *team*." Winning requires excellent communication among the players in order to ensure a coordinated effort and optimal performance.

Each player must fulfill his or her office or purpose effectively in order for the team to succeed. A team with a great defense but poor offense is a losing team. The same can be said about a team with a great offense and poor defense. All successful sports teams work on constantly improving their communication during the game in order to better handle the challenges they face and overcome them.

In summary, coordination plays a key role in the success of any organism and for that matter, any organization. Harmony in the organism is created when all its parts are fulfilling their purpose and office. The innate intelligence of the body coordinates all. The vehicle that it uses is the nervous system. Optimal coordination therefore requires that all parts of the organism are intact and communicating clearly. Chiropractic focuses solely on optimizing that communication by reducing vertebral subluxations' obstruction of nerve function. Therefore, it is the chiropractic adjustment that helps to restore the optimal coordination and harmonious function among the parts.

BJ Palmer

• • •

Time always has and always will perpetuate those methods which better serve mankind. Chiropractic is no exception.

My illustrious father placed this trust in my keeping, to keep it pure and unsullied or defamed. I pass it on to you unstained, to protect as he would have you do. As he passed on, so will I. We admonish you to keep this principle and practice unadulterated and unmixed. Humanity needed then what he gave us.

You need now what I give you.

Out there in those great open spaces are multitudes seeking what you possess. The burdens are heavy; responsibilities are many; obligations are providential; but the satisfaction of traveling the populated highways and byways, relieving suffering and adding millions of years to lives of millions of people, will bring forth satisfaction and glories with greater blessings than you think.

Time is of the essence.

May God flow from above down His bounteous strengths, courage, and understanding to carry on; and may your Innates receive and act on that free flow of wisdom from above down, inside out… for you have in your possession a sacred trust.

Guard it well.

PRINCIPLE 33

The Law of Demand and Supply
Lacy Book, DC, and Shawn Dill, DC

● ● ●

The law of demand and supply is existent in the body in its ideal state, wherein the "clearinghouse" is the brain, innate intelligence the virtuous "banker," brain cells "clerks," and nerve cells "messengers."

WHEN WE WERE INITIALLY TASKED with attempting to tackle principle 33, we have to admit that we were not necessarily jumping up and down with joy.

The law of demand and supply is a very difficult principle to tackle. We have often considered that the number 33 is such a significant number that our forebears set out to outline thirty-three principles but came up one short and threw in the law of demand and supply! They even screwed with the name—who calls it "demand and supply"?

One of the reasons we feel that they intentionally used "demand and supply," rather than the conventional "supply and demand" was to highlight and illustrate how our Chiropractic philosophy is different than the traditional "outside-in" view of the world.

As we begin this discussion, it is important to highlight that the law of demand and supply describes the relationship that occurs between the tissue cell and the innate intelligence via the normal complete cycle.

The "demand" comes from innate intelligence and is placed on the tissue cells. The "supply" also comes from innate intelligence, which must supply the tissue cell with its needs to carry out its primary function in maintaining the coordination and health of the entire organism.

Therefore, when communicating this concept with the general public, it is important to communicate that health is entirely dependent upon the law of demand and supply. As life occurs, health is maintained through the state of coordination in the body. Coordination is achieved through the law of demand and supply.

Innate intelligence runs the show. It places demands on the cells that they must respond to in order to maintain health. It supplies the tissue cells with nutrients, materials, and forces so that they can respond to its demands. If the law of demand and supply is broken in any way, the health of the organism is compromised.

The job of the chiropractor is to ensure that the law of demand and supply is present and fully satisfied at all times.

As we begin to move the discussion more into the realm of chiropractic practice, we need to expand upon the concepts.

The tissue cells of every patient are constantly sending information to the innate intelligence concerning their state and well-being. This information is sent as impressions over the afferent nerve to the brain.

Stephenson refers to the brain as the clearinghouse. A clearinghouse is defined as a central agency for the collection, classification, and distribution, especially of information. This is a fantastic analogy and way of viewing the brain's role in receiving and processing the impressions from the tissue cells along with the processing of the resulting mental impulses that are subsequently sent back to the tissue cells.

If the brain is the clearinghouse, then it simply serves as a collection and distribution point. The actual thinking and decision making occur at the hands of innate intelligence. As such, innate intelligence becomes the true source of the demand and supply.

For that reason, Stephenson refers to innate intelligence as the "banker." The banker receives and distributes money or currency. The currency in this case is incoming impressions from tissue cells and outgoing mental impulses from the brain cells.

Because the brain cells are distributing the mental impulses from the banker, they are referred to as the "clerks." They dispatch the mental impulses from innate intelligence through the efferent nerve to the tissue cell.

This is why the nerve cells are called "messengers." They dispatch the impressions from the tissue cells and deliver the mental impulses from the brain cells.

From a chiropractic-practice standpoint, it is critical that the "currency exchange" is free of interference. If the impressions are altered or if the transmission of the mental impulse is interfered with, this can disrupt the law of demand and supply and result in the incoordination of dis-ease.

In order to see this principle in action, you simply need to visit any chiropractor's office around the world. Not only will you see the law of demand and supply in the patients and practice members, but you can also see this at work when you see mothers and their children in the office.

A mother is constantly attentive to the signs and signals of her baby. When the baby cries, this signals to the mother that there is a need, and she seeks to answer that need.

However, the mother is the one who places the demand on the baby. The baby cries. It does not ask for nutrition, comfort, and so on. The mother knows what is best and places that demand on the baby. Simultaneous to that, the mother must supply the baby with its needs.

In conclusion, we can experience the law of demand and supply in our practices as we attempt to reach more people with the chiropractic story.

When we look out at the world, we see sick and confused people who have bought into a failing philosophy of health.

Sick and suffering humanity constantly sends us signs (impressions) that they have a need. As chiropractors, we act like a clearinghouse. The principles of chiropractic act as the banker, constantly charging us with the *demand* to communicate the principles to the world. The principles of chiropractic also *supply* us with the tools to communicate the principles to the world.

Our marketing of our message through various media serves as the clerk. As individual chiropractors, we are the messengers.

In the end, the law of demand and supply not only determines how our patients or practice members respond to our care but also how the world responds to our message.

Get it right, and the world will be a better place.

Bonus: Blue Ocean Marketing Strategy for Chiropractic
Andreas Söderström, DC, ACP

• • •

Chiropractic Principles as a Strategy to Differentiate in the Market Universe

Recognition of the fact that chiropractic is viewed as a part of a broader commodity market has driven this insight to investigate and compare known business strategies with the principles and philosophy of chiropractic for understanding the position of chiropractic as a profession in the market universe. Researching this topic has demonstrated certain risks when chiropractic is forced to fit into a set market and revealed certain benefits for the profession to align with its core values. The discussion expresses the importance for chiropractic to create compelling value for the users. I also consider ideas for the future of chiropractic.

In most societies with a health-care system, chiropractic is categorized as one profession among many others in the same market, relieving mainly low-back pain. Outside the market, people refer to "back crackers" with the association of pain. Other professions claiming they are doing the same thing may be physiotherapy, acupuncture, medicine, and even massage therapy.

In contrast, traditional straight chiropractic philosophy is not based on the treatment of spinal pain and disability or other symptomatic presentations. Is it instead the philosophy of chiropractic that will make it differentiate in the market universe? How could chiropractic use that as a strategy for future market position? Furthermore, what market forces are driving chiropractic, and how does the consumer know the difference between the different professions? How does the market universe view this question? What is the difference?

Market Universe

W. Chan Kim and Renée Morgan in *Blue Ocean Strategy* (Harvard Business School Publishing Corporation, 2005) explain that you may imagine the market universe being composed of two sorts of oceans: red oceans and blue oceans. Red oceans are the known market spaces and represent all the industries in existence today. Blue oceans are the unknown market spaces, which include all the industries not in existence today.

Red Ocean

Industry boundaries, regulations, and rules are defined and accepted in the red oceans. The competitive rules of the game are known in this market. Here companies try to grab a greater share of existing demand by outperforming their rivals or by winning the game. For the past few decades, the field of business strategy has been dominated by a focus on value capture through competitive strategy, largely under the influence of Michael Porter, Porter, and Michael E. in *Competitive Strategy* (New York: The Free Press, 1980). As the market space of red oceans gets busy and crowded, prospects for profits and growth are reduced. Products become commodities, and cutthroat competition turns the red ocean bloody. Hence the term *red oceans* may be used. With this concept in mind, one may look at medicine as a big white shark and chiropractic as a salmon swimming upstream in the red ocean.

The red-ocean strategy is as follows:

- Compete in existing market spaces.
- Beat the competition.
- Exploit existing demand.
- Make the value-cost trade-off.

- Align the whole system of a firm's activities with its strategic choice of differentiation or low cost.

Commodity Market

Commoditization occurs as a goods or services market loses differentiation across its supply base either by a surplus or simply by copying. Commodities are things of value, of uniform quality, that are produced by many different producers; the items from each different producer are considered equivalent or alternatives. Today, chiropractic is seen as one of many other professions that deal with spinal pain and therefore part of a commodity market. Similar businesses become a commodity mainly because they are similar, according to Kjell A. Nordström and Jonas Ridderstråle in *Funky Business* (Bookhouse Publishing, 1999). They call this a surplus society, where a "surplus of similar companies, employing similar people, with similar educational backgrounds, coming up with similar ideas, producing similar things, with similar prices, and similar quality" will create a commodity market. A commodity has full or partial fungibility—that is, the market treats its instances as equivalent or nearly so with no regard for who produces or delivers them.

Unfortunately, from the customer's point of view, he or she cannot be sure any longer what kind of chiropractic care to receive when choosing from the commodity market. Still, most people seeking, for example, a dentist for a tooth problem expect and will find a dentist who will examine the teeth. The consumers in this case are not confused on what care to receive. In contrast, there is now a wide range of care offered from most chiropractors when someone is seeking chiropractic attention. The user many times feels confused about what chiropractic is based on what they receive.

In reality, it will always be important to navigate successfully in the red ocean by outcompeting rivals. Many of the practice-building companies within chiropractic are basically working with this fact. They teach their clients how to be seen and heard in the red ocean and how to compete with others in that market. Red oceans will always matter and will always be a fact of business life and present in any community with an opinion.

I believe many chiropractors are drawn into the known market where they think they need to compete or add value to the consumer by adding modalities to their scope of practice, such as laser therapy, acupuncture, nutrition, massage, and even the use of prescription drugs, as desired by many chiropractors. Chiropractic may fit into the variety of different therapies when its objective is limited to condition-centered care primarily directed at treating pain. However, as the service-commodity market regarding taking care of pain gets more crowded, competing for a share of contracting markets, the message gets even further confused and diluted and quality may go down at the same time.

Other Factors Driving Chiropractic toward a Commodity Market

As Kenneth Hudson stated in 1978 in *The Jargon of Professions*, "If one wished to kill a profession, to remove its cohesion and its strength, the most effective way would be to forbid the use of its characteristic language." The language or the terminology of chiropractic is flooded with medical terminology and short selling its own lexicon, which is driving chiropractic further toward an allopathic model of care.

The Early Fights for the Principle of Chiropractic

In the spring of 1906, D. D. Palmer would be the first of thousands of chiropractors who would go to jail for chiropractic. This occurred for three-quarters of the century. Herbert C. Hender, DC, states that "from early days, this man saw the necessity of banding together sincere men who had courage of their convictions, into a national group for the purpose of defense and protection. From the beginning of the old U.C.A. to date, more than 19,000 cases have been defended, under his guidance, in every state, province, and many foreign countries, from police courts to supreme courts, winning so consistently that such trials now are practically stopped."[5] Hender is referring to the enormous work from B. J. Palmer.

The early chiropractors dedicated their lives to fighting for chiropractic, and I dare say they reconstructed the world by introducing and developing a new paradigm. Over 120 years later, since the first jailing, it appears that the fighting has been going on for so long that most of the profession has forgotten what the early pioneers were fighting for. Legislation in numerous states and nations has attempted to expand the scope of practice even to introduce prescription rights. This has taken the chiropractic profession far away from its core value and main objective and deep into a commodity market. Therefore, we need to remember our history and realize it is time for a professional renaissance consistent with the core values of chiropractic. Clearly big, successful chiropractic practices globally understand and show how the market values chiropractic without the introduction of other modalities with increased costs.

Could it be as easy as focusing on the main objective of chiropractic to differentiate it in the commodity market? The best strategy is a simple one, commonly known as the Grandma test: "If your grandma understands the core compelling value and philosophy without explanation, you have a good strategy."

Blue Oceans

Kim and Mauuborgne show that in contrast to red oceans, blue oceans are defined by market spaces not yet explored, which demand creation and therefore offer the opportunity for highly profitable growth. Although blue oceans may be created well beyond existing industry boundaries, most are created from within red oceans by expanding and exploring existing industry boundaries. Competition in blue oceans is irrelevant because the rules of the game are not set, and therefore, there is no game to be won. The term *blue ocean* is a great analogy to describe market space that is vast,

---

5 Herbert C. Hender, quoted in B. J. Palmer, *The Bigness of the Fellow Within*, vol. 22 (Prague: The Palmer School of Chiropractic, 1949), xviii.

deep, and not explored. The potential in blue oceans is wide and with no boundaries.

The blue oceans strategy is as follows:

- Create uncontested market space.
- Make the competition irrelevant.
- Create and capture new demand.
- Break the value-cost trade-off.
- Align the whole system of a firm's activities in pursuit of differentiation and low cost.

The early chiropractors were not fighting for the right to add drugs, surgery, exercise, laser therapy, or any other modality into the practice of chiropractic. Instead, they were fighting for a principle to help humanity. The attitude and drive coming from the founder of chiropractic, D. D. Palmer, then his son, B. J. Palmer, and followed by others, focused on a truth developed from the philosophy of chiropractic, and this very attitude and drive are what make it difficult for chiropractic to be dictated into a market with a different paradigm. The hallmark of that paradigm is its condition-centered objectives, which are inconsistent with the vertebral-subluxation-centered objectives, rendering the chiropractic profession divided and not united as a profession. As posted by Joe Strauss on January 31, 2014, "The medical objective is to treat, cure, prevent disease, its causes and effect by whatever means necessary or effective (drugs or drugless, allopathic or homeopathic, chemical or natural). That's why the medical profession had so much opposition to D. D. Palmer's idea from the start and why B. J. Palmer makes no mention of disease in the thirty-three principles. If the chiropractic and the medical professions could have understood that one simple difference, we would have saved one-hundred-plus years of conflict between those who wanted to affect the matter (the medical objective) and those who wanted to remove an interference to the force (the chiropractic objective)."

From a business-strategy point of view, the early fight and crusader-like attitude in chiropractic come close to what is referred to as a

33

reconstructionist view of strategy. Interestingly, there are similar characteristics across blue-ocean creations. In contrast to companies playing by traditional rules, the creators of blue oceans never used the competition as their benchmark. Instead, they made it irrelevant by creating a leap in value for both buyers and the company itself. Other examples of this are when personal computers replaced the typewriter or when the traditional film camera was replaced with the new digital technology. This created a new market with no competition left. Companies like the world-leading camera manufacturer Hasselblad almost disappeared when they refused to use the new digital technology.

While the competition-based red-ocean strategy assumes that an industry's structural conditions are given and that firms are forced to compete within them, blue-ocean strategy is based on the view that market boundaries, rules, and structure are not given and can be reconstructed by the actions and beliefs of the creators. This is called the reconstructionist view. In the red ocean, differentiation costs because firms compete with the same best practice rule, like many chiropractors traditionally have been doing. Companies, in this case chiropractors, can either create greater value to customers at a higher cost or create reasonable value at a lower cost. In other words, strategy is essentially a choice between differentiation and low cost.

Many chiropractors add modalities to a greater cost in order to create a differentiation in the commodity market, and this is clearly seen by the way marketing is done.

In the reconstructionist world, however, the strategic aim is to create new rules for the game by breaking the existing value and cost trade-off and thereby creating a blue ocean. Recognizing that structure and market boundaries exist only in managers' minds, practitioners who hold the reconstructionist view do not let existing market structures limit their thinking. They see that the demand is out there, largely untapped. This is when chiropractors should shift the focus and vision toward the belief that every man, woman, and child deserves to be checked for vertebral subluxation. This, in turn, requires a shift of attention from supply to demand, from a focus on competing to a focus on leaving the competition behind or not even recognizing them as competition.

This creation of blue oceans is driving costs down while simultaneously driving value up for buyers. In chiropractic, this will happen when people value the product of chiropractic from its main objective, which is to check for vertebral subluxations and get adjusted when necessary. This is how a leap in value for both the chiropractor or company and its buyers is achieved. Because buyer value comes from the utility and price that the company offers to buyers and because the value to the company is generated from price and cost structure, blue-ocean strategy is achieved only when the whole system of the company's utility, price, and cost activities is properly aligned. Blue-ocean strategy integrates the range of a firm's functional and operational activities. In this sense, blue-ocean strategy is more than innovation. It is about strategy that embraces the entire system of a company's activities.

A philosophy is a system a person performs for the conduct of life, the theory, and the morality one chose as a guide in life. The philosophy in chiropractic puts forth the theory of chiropractic and gives answers to why. The science of chiropractic tests the theory and that is done by the application, the art. Chiropractic philosophy differs in its main objective in the crowded commodity market where all is similar.

The definition of chiropractic by Stephenson 1927 is the following: "Chiropractic is the philosophy science and art of things natural, a system of adjusting the segments of the spinal column by hand only, for the correction of the cause of dis-ease."

By definition, a profession is a group of individuals professing an idea. According to Joe Strauss, "The idea of chiropractic is that of removing interference to the full expression of the forces of the innate intelligence of the body. It is not about changing symptoms, changing the world, or changing anything else. It is about removing nerve interference and allowing to happen what is going to happen."

This is done by locating, analyzing, and adjusting vertebral subluxations. The strategy to do this is by "ensuring access to vertebral subluxation correction for all people during all stages of life regardless of the presence or absence of symptoms. Both chiropractic and the vertebral subluxation have been defined by the founders, and therefore no organization or individual has the authority to change the definition, or objective of the profession. Using the business strategy previously described and linking that with the objective of chiropractic, it is clear to me that the practice of chiropractic should not be placed into a market with known boundaries from the perspective of symptom relief. From a philosophy standpoint, it has no concern for chiropractic.

Chiropractic could shift the whole focus on how to differentiate in a set market. The market is wide open like a blue ocean for the purpose of correcting vertebral subluxations regardless of conditions or symptoms. If we as chiropractors can communicate that to the consumers and they value what chiropractic is about, it opens up a limitless market. However, if we as a profession continue to embrace a condition-centered scope of practice with the primary purpose of removing pain, we choose to compete with all other therapies claiming the same in the commodity market.

The Importance of Considering the Market

Like I stated earlier, you will always have a red ocean, and that strategy is actually helping and showing us how to differ. Chiropractic can use this information and by observing what is happening in the commodity market find a different path or strategy for future chiropractic. This is something to be grateful for, and this is what is giving us clues on how to proceed by navigating with the help of chiropractic principles. How could chiropractic differentiate and prosper in future markets?

What if the public understood that the role of the chiropractor is the removal of the vertebral subluxation to restore optimal regulation of the body's adaptability? What if chiropractic as a profession worked in the practice of salutogenesis rather than pathogenesis? According to the salutogenic perspective, each person should engage in health-promoting actions to cause health while they secondarily benefit from the prevention of disease and infirmity. Pathogenesis, in contrast, in a complementary fashion, primarily focuses on prevention of disease and infirmity, with a secondary benefit of health promotion. Both models assume if the primary focus is attained, the secondary purpose will follow."

What if the mission of chiropractic was to adjust every man, woman, and child who values getting adjusted for a vertebral subluxation when indicated for the removal of interference and therefore optimal regulation of the body's adaptability? The vision would be for chiropractic to create a compelling value for every man, woman, and child to use chiropractic as an integrated part of their lives. This would change the focus and the target group for chiropractic within the market universe.

The situation for chiropractic is that all providers of care are in a contested market space—a red ocean.

A complication is that a lot of the strong forces in the red ocean are pushing chiropractic away from its core values and therefore chiropractic reasons. If you can't beat them, join them. So chiropractic over time switches over to an allopathic paradigm with the thinking it will grow stronger. But the very opposite may happen since the chiropractic message will get so diluted that it will stop existing and be consumed by the allopathic message. The consumer gets confused and finds no compelling value in seeking chiropractic care. The chiropractic profession starts losing its identity. I propose that by establishing an uncontested market space where only chiropractic exists, applying the understanding of chiropractic principles to differentiate it in the commodity market through the compelling value of the focus on locating, analyzing, and adjusting when necessary the vertebral subluxation, chiropractic will prosper in the future.

Thomas A. Gelardi, DC, states, "If the solution does not come from within the profession, it will come from outside forces. If it does not come from the highest principles, it probably will not come at all, and the wolves at the door will feast."

Andreas Soderstrom, DC, ACP

> **You never know how far reaching something you think,
> say, or do will affect the lives of millions tomorrow.**
>
> —B. J. Palmer, DC

ACKNOWLEDGMENTS

• • •

I WANT TO THANK YOU for participating in this journey. My hope is that this body of work brings about and discussion, questions, and insights for yourself and our great profession so that we can continue to evolve the philosophy, science, and art of chiropractic. My wife, Gabriela, gave me the initial idea, and she is always loving and supportive of my endeavors and chiropractic. For her, I am forever grateful.

I want to thank each and every person who contributed to this book. The authors were gracious and precise with my deadlines and enthusiastic to participate. My good friend Boo Burnier gave me the idea for the title, and I thank him for his genius. I will begin to have this book translated into other languages and donate a portion of the profit back to chiropractic causes.

Thank you,
David Serio, Doctor of Chiropractic
Buenos Aires, Argentina, 2017

For more information about Dr. David Serio or to contact him, visit his website at www.davidseriodc.com.

ABOUT THE AUTHOR

• • •

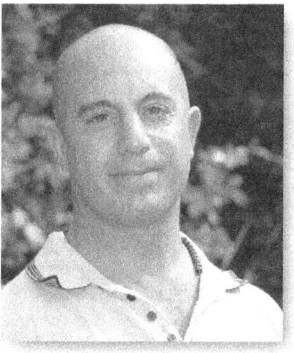

Dr. David Serio graduated from the Sherman College of Straight Chiropractic in December 1999 and founded Vida Chiropractic in 2000 in Buenos Aires, Argentina.

An international speaker and teacher, Serio is the creator of the Vida Chiropractic seminars series, the Life Evolution experience and Life Evolution Coaching. He is a husband and father and resides in Buenos Aires, Argentina.

Dr. David Serio can be contacted at www.Davidseriodc.com.

www.ingramcontent.com/pod-product-compliance
Lightning Source LLC
Chambersburg PA
CBHW050052230526
45470CB00004B/1491